Anti-Aging Dentistry

Anti-Aging Dentistry

Restoring Youth, One Smile at a Time

Dr. Kourosh Maddahi

Copyright © 2014 by Dr. Kourosh Maddahi

All rights reserved. This work may not be translated or copied in whole or in part without the written permission of the author except for brief excerpts in connection with reviews or scholarly analysis. Use in connection with any form of information storage and retrieval, electronic adaptation, computer software, or by similar or dissimilar methodology now known or hereafter developed is forbidden.

The use in this publication of trade names, trademarks, service marks and similar terms, even if they are not identified as such, is not to be taken as an expression of opinion as to whether or not they are subject to proprietary rights. The Publisher is not associated with any product mentioned in this book.

This publication is designed to provide accurate and authoritative information in regard to the subject matter covered at the time of publication. It is sold on the understanding that the Publisher is not engaged in rendering professional services. If professional advice or other expert assistance is required regarding any subject matter covered in this book, the services of a competent professional should be sought.

ISBN: 978-0-9916252-0-8

Printed in the United States of America

To my Father, who gave me the gift of logic; my Mother, who gave me the gift of compassion; my Wife, who gave me the gift of support; and my Children, who gave me the gift of endurance.

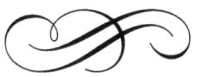

Table of Contents

Preface	1
Chapter 1 | What is Anti-Aging Dentistry	7
Chapter 2 | Meet Dr. Maddahi	11
Chapter 3 | Clenching and Grinding	27
Chapter 4 | Food and Habits	35
Chapter 5 | Support from Inside	47
Chapter 6 | Technology	59
Chapter 7 | Pain Free Dentistry	67
Chapter 8 | Dentistry from the Outside In: Case Studies	71
Chapter 9 | Tetracycline Stains	81
Chapter 10 | Quality of Life	87
Chapter 11 | Self Evaluation	95
Closing Note	113

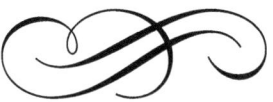

Preface

By Caroline Dupuy Heerwagen

I consider myself a pretty average adult woman in America. I worry about men, I cry during romantic comedies, and I love Haagen Dazs. I'm not a super model, but I'm not terrible looking, and despite my love for ice cream, I try and work out and eat right to keep my body from doing something that is known in my family as Heerwagen hips (that might seem funny, but trust me, the threat is real and terrifying). I do my best to stay looking my best, but no matter what I do the fact remains that I'm getting older, and I'm starting to notice things about my face and body that I have never noticed before, and honestly, I can't say I'm thrilled about any of them.

I say I think these qualities make me average because I've done the research. I know that I'm not alone in any of it. In fact, I recently read a study conducted on women across the country by NBC News that reported over 97% of the women taking part in the study came back with at least one "I hate the way I look" moment during the course of a day. In fact, according to a poll on over 300 women by Glamour magazine (of all sources) about the psychology of the typical adult, most early 20s to late 40s American ladies have their attention on the way they look in a negative way anywhere from 13 to 100 times a day.

I don't have to state it, but I will: this figure is depressing because it points right to the fact that we, as a society, are completely obsessed with our appearances, and more often times than not, we're not happy about what we see. When examining this I think it's clear that what's happening is we're not satisfied with our looks because we're constantly faced with pop culture, the media, and Hollywood telling us we should be a size 0 and have flawless skin. What's worse, those kinds of impossible standards are designed to seem achievable, even though they're really not for most of us, leaving a sort of "what am I doing wrong?" feeling in their wake. I mean, honestly, I read an article the other day that Scarlett Johansson looks terrible now because she was spotted with cellulite while on some beach, as if cellulite is something no one should be allowed to have. Did you know 80-90% of women have cellulite? Women who don't get enough food to eat in Africa have cellulite. This standard is ridiculous.

From our haircuts to the cars we drive, the way someone sees us seems so important that it has become what our entire social structure is based around. You're only cool if you dress a certain way and your facial structure closely resembles either half of Brangelina. We get older, and this desperate situation transforms from a preference to a terrified fight against time and everything that she wishes upon us.

In light of this all-encompassing subject, I pose the question: what does the common person really know about the ever expanding field of anti-aging?

The term all on its own is interesting, because it means, in theory, that one is opposed to aging. I think pretty much anyone can relate to feeling this way, but as we all know, it's a rather silly thing to be adverse to because absolutely no matter what any one of us does we *are* going to age. We're going to look and feel older, because we're going to *be* older. Nonetheless, we fight the good fight, for better or worse, against the inevitable. We use creams, pump our bodies full of all the latest in health trends, and exhaust ourselves with work-out regimens to keep our abs flat, our skin smooth, and our prayers alive that everything else will just… defy gravity.

The thing is, for as many square inches of our bodies that we don't want to look a day over the legal drinking age, there are about 50 different theories trending that claim to be the cure for the years that are passing. Amateurs develop most of these "cures" with no actual experience doing anything but perfecting their yoga moves. That may seem harsh, but at the end of the day, in the quest for eternal youth, it's pretty difficult to know which combination of juicing and Pilates is going to work best and where the information that you're getting on either is actually coming from.

I became recently addicted to the idea of somehow being able to find out the real truth from people who were at the top of their fields and then collecting all of this information into one place to be given to the part of the population who really want to know that kind of thing (which, if I'm going off the aforementioned studies, is most of it).

This is when I started working with a magazine called Masters of Aesthetics. I had been discussing doing some writing for the high-end beauty magazine with the creator of it, and after a few conversations, my immense curiosity on the Anti-Aging aspect of things landed me in front of Dr. Kourosh Maddahi, DDS, a dentist who was making a lot of noise in the field of Anti-Aging. At first I thought what a lot of people think when they hear the term Anti-Aging Dentistry (as the subfield has been dubbed), which was, "what?"

Subsequently what I learned about anti-aging from Dr. Maddahi was more than I learned on the subject from any other professional in the industry. He also ended up being one of the coolest, most forward-thinking guys I've ever met. So I started hanging out with Dr. Maddahi at his offices quite a bit to learn about what he was developing and how performing what is known as a "full mouth reconstruction" can change someone's entire face, giving them the same benefits that a facelift would give without having to go under the knife to get them.

I became so fascinated by the concepts that he was explaining to me that I proposed a book about it, and that's what we have now. A book. A book about the dentist who is not just attempting to make your teeth whiter, he's attempting to take ten years of aging off your face. It resulted in an entire sub-field of dentistry that is now catching fire throughout both the dental and cosmetic world. That ain't bad.

From what I have gotten from Dr. Maddahi, it seems a lot of his competitors are jumping on his bandwagon. He even handed me an article in a local Beverly Hills magazine on two dentists in the San Fernando Valley who were claiming the idea as their own. None of that really comes as a surprise to Dr. Maddahi, but what most of these guys don't understand is how the hell the idea came about in the first place, which also stops them from really being able to practice it with much success.

"Most people think cosmetic dentistry is just about getting your teeth whiter," Dr. Maddahi explained to me over his large conference table, where he can be found in-between patients, hunched over whichever one of his many side projects he has going at any given hour of any given day, like developing a new mouthwash with Dead Sea Salt. In fact, with his fingers in about 5 fully functioning companies that he was instrumental in, if not solely responsible for creating, it's hard to understand how someone so busy could still maintain the kind of unwavering calm that he does every minute of every hour that I have spent with him. It's part of why if you become one of his patients, no other dentist will ever do. This leaves his office manager playing concierge more often than not, giving recommendations and dealing with all kinds of flight arrangements and accommodations for clients who now live out of town but refuse to go anywhere else.

"I spent so much time watching my patients age over the last three decades that I started to notice how their teeth affected the way they looked. This is not something most of the doctors in my field have recognized in the past. The teeth support the cheeks, the lips, and the area around the nose, which are the areas that, as years go by, start to hollow out and cause us to look older. So I started to play with the idea of using the best porcelain veneers and crowns available to counteract this."

This is a concept I had never heard of, and I don't think I'm alone in that. Even in cosmetic dentistry this idea of using veneers and crowns as a corrective method for things like straightening and adjusting the bite has only become acceptable over the last decade or so, and when Dr. Maddahi started trying to push the envelope in this direction the lab technicians that were commissioned to design the porcelain teeth for him refused to even do it. They were too worried that it would not work, and the patient would end up having more problems than they started with.

Dr. Maddahi, then a young doctor out of USC, didn't care what they said. He was sure that he could use veneers and crowns to not only straighten people's teeth, eliminating the need for braces in some cases, but also improve the shape of someone's lips and cheeks, peeling years off their faces.

He was finally able to convince one of the top lab technicians in the world to do this for him after putting his own job on the line if it didn't work as a sort of collateral. He ended up being right, making the use of veneers and crowns an acceptable alternative to braces for adults. Still, it wasn't really the advancement alone that thrilled him; it was the other part of it that he found more interesting, the fact that he was able to push something farther than anyone thought he could. This quality is the one that has allowed him to pave the way for this field of Anti-Aging Dentistry as much as he has, putting him at the forefront of the subject's development, pushing it in all new directions of speed and efficiency, landing him features on Extra TV! and CBS News to show just how much these procedures can do and how much time they strip from his patient's faces.

These results are remarkable. They give someone the most natural looking lift I have ever seen, because what he's doing is providing support from inside someone's mouth. He's not cutting and pulling back someone's skin. He's not injecting anything into it either. What he is doing is providing the skin with the support it needs to smooth out and stay that way for a very long time. This is why people look 10 to 20 years younger when he's done. They've regained their youthful smile, and their skin is smooth without being stretched. This is the stuff aging women's dreams are made of. This is the answer to where so many of these previously irreversible wrinkles that show up around one's mouth come from and how to get rid of them. This is where "anti-aging" is going. It's going towards a dentist's chair.

Chapter 1

What Is Anti-Aging Dentistry?

Dr. Maddahi has built a reputation as one of the most trusted names in cosmetic and restorative dentistry over his 27 years of practice. He has now stepped into a newly created subfield of dentistry that focuses on reversing and preventing the signs of aging that have been traced to issues arising in tooth and jaw structures. With this subfield have come breakthrough discoveries and procedures to handle them. Holding firm at the top of this field, Dr. Maddahi explains its development and its benefits.

§

When I graduated from USC Dental School in 1987, my goal was to be the best cosmetic dentist in Beverly Hills. After some years of practicing in the 90210 zip code, I started to realize that there were some holes in cosmetic dentistry that no one seemed to have the answers for.

It wasn't enough for me to just make someone's teeth whiter and straighter, and unfortunately this is about where the field stops. I knew there was more I could do for my patients. There had to be ways to give them smiles that were not just straight and white, but were structurally sound and, most of all, age-defying.

On top of that, I was convinced that the technology being used needed a huge thrust into the future to make these procedures both fast and virtually painless. The dental world needed a facelift (pun intended).

Over half the dentists in the country still use Amalgam fillings, which means that over half the people getting fillings are also being exposed to mercury vapor every time they drink something hot. This, to me, is unacceptable. And so too is the approach that many of my colleagues have to everything from anesthesia to X-Rays.

In this book I intend to explain what *can* be done in dentistry to reverse years of wear and tear, not just in someone's mouth but also to the entire bottom 1/3 of the face. This approach to dentistry is so far beyond what is being done in the field that "cosmetic dentistry" as a term no longer seemed to fit, and so Anti-Aging Dentistry was born, which is exactly what it sounds like, Dentistry that reverses or stops age.

The way this is done is through the use of porcelain veneers and crowns. These have been the backbone of cosmetic dentistry as well, but with Anti-Aging Dentistry they are being utilized in a completely unique and revolutionary way.

Typically when one needs a veneer or a crown, a dentist will shave down the tooth and adhere porcelain in the exact height and width that the tooth was previously. They might change the shape of it a bit, but that's about it. This has been accepted as the only way to really use veneers and crowns for years. However, they can do much more than this, and in this book I will reveal everything they can do.

My first discovery was in 1992. I had the idea that porcelain veneers and crowns could be used to straighten teeth. There was a huge amount of push back to this idea initially. Other dentists in the field did not like it, and I couldn't even get any of the lab technicians (the guys who actually make the veneers and crowns) to work with me on this theory.

The reason for this is because in dental school you're taught that the last thing you want to do is remove unnecessary tooth structure because the more of the original bone you take away the weaker the tooth will be. That is partially true, but it is also just as true that there are ways to protect teeth. I knew that if I could get one of the lab technicians to make the porcelain veneers and crowns for me, I could also ensure that they stayed in someone's mouth for a long time.

It took a lot of convincing for me to finally get a lab technician that I thought could do a good job to construct the pieces the way I wanted them. I was going to be shaving down more of the tooth than was generally accepted as workable, so that I could put on crowns and veneers that were straighter than the original teeth were. No one had done this, and there was a chance it wouldn't work.

In the end it did work, and even though it took a lot of convincing for many years each time I wanted to do this kind of work, eventually this became a more acceptable way of approaching a case. Now using veneers and crowns to straighten teeth is not completely unheard of, though it is still viewed by some as unorthodox.

This was the first step in pushing the boundaries on what veneers and crowns could do, and it's been evolving ever since. We've now discovered that we can use these pieces to give someone support in the lower 1/3 of the face where it had been missing, thus giving someone a complete lift and peeling many years from their face.

In short, this is a new and exciting way to approach Anti-Aging. It's long-lasting, it's virtually pain free, and there's no recovery time.

I have seen patients who have felt they were never going to be able to smile, beam. I have seen wrinkles that were deemed impossible to get rid of, vanish and watched 20 years fall off of someone's face in just a week.

Anti-Aging Dentistry is filling the holes I'd spotted so many years ago, and I'm happy to say the world of dentistry will never be the same.

5 Ways Veneers and Crowns Can Change a Smile

- Provide support to the lips and cheeks
- Reshape teeth to complement one's face shape
- Open up a collapsed bite
- Correct discoloration
- Straighten crooked teeth

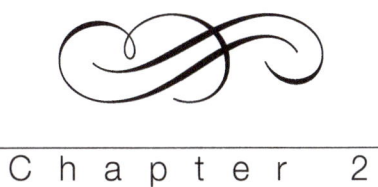

Chapter 2
Meet Dr. Maddahi

An introduction to the man behind the "cutting-edge" of Anti-Aging Dentistry by Caroline Dupuy Heerwagen.

§

There's probably no one I've met who is looking for the challenge more than Dr. Maddahi. From what I've been able to observe, it's what keeps him moving everyday. He's never satisfied and doesn't even understand people who are.

"Most people I talk to say that when work is stressful that's when they have the hardest time. I find it's the opposite for me. I thrive in those times. It's harder for me to be on vacation or even relax on the weekends. I simply love my work, and I'm happiest when I'm producing something. That's what gets me going. I never want to be done pushing myself to the limits."

When Dr. Maddahi discovered that he was right about being able to straighten teeth with veneers and crowns, and this started to become a more common tool in the industry, it was the speed with which it could be done that he started to focus on.

He realized that often times the kinds of people who would seek him out were the best in their fields of business or entertainment.

These types of people really don't have very much time to get procedures like this done, but they were desperate for the work and would implore him to find a way to make it happen.

Most dentists would have turned these cases away, saying a full mouth of veneers and crowns (also known as a full mouth reconstruction) would take over a month, and the patient had better come back when they had that kind of time. Dr. Maddahi knew this could not be, and he set out to find a way to make these procedures much faster.

How much faster? You can be in and out of his chair in as little time as a week. This seemed impossible to me when he told me. That's over 75% faster.

"Let me explain," he said to me, all grinning and proud. "There are a few things that have gotten me to this point when it comes to speed.

"There's a test that one is required to take before applying to dental school called the DAT (Dental Aptitude Test). It has all the usual questions you'd expect about biology, math, and all of that, but there is also this one section called 'Spatial Symmetry' and there's really nothing you could do to learn more about this subject or why it's there.

"I didn't really understand the point of it myself, but when I got my results back I was in the top 1% for this section in the country. It's not even something you can practice."

"What *is* Spatial Symmetry?" I asked.

"Basically you're given shapes and asked to figure out how they fit into each other and how they work together, but because you're given so little time, you can't draw anything. You have to be able to construct things, play with shapes, and fit shapes together in your mind. That's the easiest way I can describe it."

"That sounds complicated."

"I think for most people it is. But I understood the subject very well. Now, after I had graduated from dental school I was talking to one of my friends in the dental field about how to fix a particular person's smile. I was able to spot what he could not rather quickly, and before I knew what was happening, it had snowballed.

"Colleagues started to come by and ask me, 'What would you do with this person?' 'What would you do with my Mom?' I was consulting people a lot and a couple of them said to me after awhile, 'How do you see these things?'

"That's when I realized what was being measured in that test. I can look at a space and construct something new there in my head without needing to physically put it there or even really look at it for very long. I saw that this was something I could do that was different.

"Now, looking at it that way, if you have an image of something in your mind, an image of how you want something to look, and then you start working backwards to how it looks in front of you, you can then start to work on techniques that will help you get to the end result quicker.

"When you don't really know what the end result could look like, and there's so much uncertainty, so much back and forth with the lab, and the lab doesn't know what you mean, and you're really guessing, every step of the process takes a lot longer. So every time I'm working on a patient I'm working based on an image in my head of exactly what it is going to look like when it is done.

"This also helps with preparation time, because I know exactly what I'm looking for when I'm preparing the teeth and what it's going to take to get the teeth to where they need to be for what I am envisioning.

"Let me give you an example. I just finished doing some work on actress Marisol Nichols. She came in to see me with this insecurity about her teeth. Marisol is a very beautiful and talented woman, but she had never been able to smile on the red carpet because she was so embarrassed about the way her teeth looked. As an actress, this was a real problem for her. She appeared more serious on camera, and she even looked older than she was.

"So I started to work on this with her. I told her how I wanted her teeth to look and we made a wax up so that she could see the end result on a model. From the start she had a concern that a lot of my clients have, which is that they don't want to have 'horse teeth'. They're worried their teeth are going to look like fake teeth.

"No one wants to look like they're wearing dentures, no matter how old they are. I can sit there and try and explain that it's not going to happen till I'm blue in the face, but most of the time, if someone is worried about this it's pretty hard to dislodge that fear until they see what their teeth will actually look like for themselves.

"As soon as we got the temporaries in her mouth everything changed. She was so elated with the temps that she started going on auditions right away, something she had been worried she was going to have to put on hold until the procedure was completely done. She was in love with her teeth! She would text me about how happy they made her. She couldn't see what I could see before that point. She hadn't been able to see the end product.

"It's something people have to see for themselves. They have to see with their own eyes what I've seen in my head in order to understand what I'm wanting for them.

"So that was the first part of it all. The second part of what makes what I do so much faster is that after I graduated in 1987 from USC all the way up to 1996 I was working in an office that had an in house lab technician."

"And that's unusual?"

"Yes, it is very rare, which is unfortunate because since he was there and I was working so closely with him, I could constantly go back and forth with him and talk about different concepts.

"I was able to gain an understanding for exactly what the limits were and how we could make things look better and move faster. It gave me a much more extensive understanding of the materials we were working with, how flexible they were, and how far we could push it.

"Since I had a technician there, I actually had so much more freedom to push the limits because I could do two sets of temporaries and see how one set worked in comparison to the other set. It gave me a huge advantage because I knew what *could* be done and what a lab technician actually *needed* in order to do quality work."

"I've heard you use a lab technician who works exclusively with you now, is that right?" I asked.

"Yes. I've been working with him for so long that he really understands what I'm looking for now.

"Many of the technicians I've worked with over my career have remarked that the cases I get are very diverse. In reality, it's just my work that varies so extremely. Every patient that sits in front of me is going to get a completely unique set of teeth because they have a completely unique face. I take everything from face shape to skin and hair color into account when I'm working on someone's smile, and this is what sets these cases apart, and makes them look so natural."

The Italian Job

"At a very early point in my career I started doing these jobs that were high profile and set me up for this kind of rapid speed and attention to detail.

"I would fly into Milan, Italy with an associate of mine and we would do about 250 crowns in 2 ½ weeks. We would have master technicians flown in from Los Angeles and Japan who would work three shifts, 24 hours a day.

"The people that we were working on were the top executives and very well known people in Italy. The work was extremely intense, and it sort of changed the game for me.

"There was no room for error, because there was no way to extend these trips. We had our practices to get back to, and the people we were working on had very busy lives, so the schedule was very tight.

"Now, I don't know how much experience you've had with situations like that…"

I laughed out loud, "Like that? None."

"Well, we found out very quickly that whatever could go wrong was not only going to go wrong, but was going to go as wrong as it possibly could go, every single trip.

"What that kind of pressure does is pretty special. It makes you able to think on your feet in a way that is hard to describe or teach anyone. It's something you have to go through. The level of necessity there to make things work is so high that you have to gain the ability (if you don't have it already) to trouble shoot and problem solve very quickly and calmly.

"You don't have the luxury of trying stuff out with the normal attitude that if it doesn't work we'll just try something else. You don't have that. There's not enough time to redo anything, so you have to get it right with what you have the first time.

"That pressure has been the number one most important thing that changed the way I work. It was a real turning point for me. It gave me the ability to quickly come up with solutions and handle cases that most people would just not know what to do with.

"That prepared me for the next phases of my career."

"You've got to be kidding me. What happened with those guys?"

"The Italy guys?"

"Yeah, the Italy guys."

"After awhile it became not worth it in a big way. I would come home and it would take me weeks to recover from the exhaustion. There was no way I would have been able to keep going."

"Why did you do it to begin with then?" I asked, knowing the answer already.

"It paid! Really well. I was young and eager to do exciting things and that was exactly what it was, until it wasn't, and then it was taking away from everything else in my life, including my practice at home and my own personal health.

"So at some point you have to say enough is enough and know that there are going to be other opportunities to do exciting things. It prepares you for the big stuff."

"Sounds like walking away from a black jack table." I was joking, but now that I think about it, it really does. Dr. Maddahi just nodded.

You Are Being Televised

The next phase Dr. Maddahi was referring to was the one where he appeared on dozens of reality TV makeover shows, which we talked about after I got to see one being filmed for Extra TV!

Actress Marisol Nichols' full mouth reconstruction was being covered for a segment on Anti-Aging Dentistry and what it can do.

I was struck by how calm Dr. Maddahi was in front of the camera. I knew that he must have done quite a few of these shows to be that comfortable.

"When did you start doing these kinds of things? You looked so relaxed, so I'm guessing you've been at it for quite some time."

"I started back in the early 2000s. In those first few years of my having my own practice I began to realize that it was very important to be connected to other professionals in related fields who were like-minded.

"So I started to create a network of dermatologists, plastic surgeons, hair and makeup artists, image consultants and everything in between so that if I needed to I could call on these people and together we could give someone a full body makeover.

"About two years later the whole concept of makeover shows started to come out, and I got a phone call one day from one of the very talented plastic surgeons I know telling me there was this patient that he thought would be an amazing candidate for a full body makeover, and that Entertainment Tonight was interested in the story.

"He asked me if I would do the teeth for it, and I said of course I would and told him to send her over to me.

Restoring Youth, One Smile at a Time

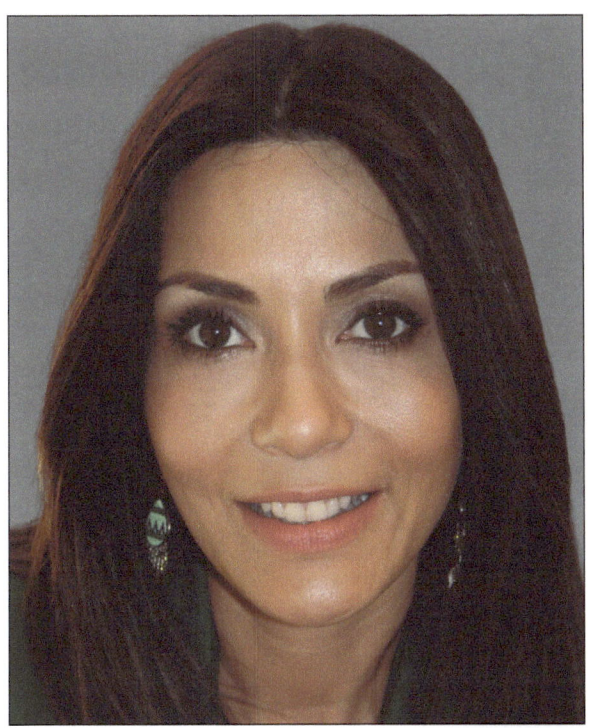

Actress Marisol Nichols Before

Actress Marisol Nichols After

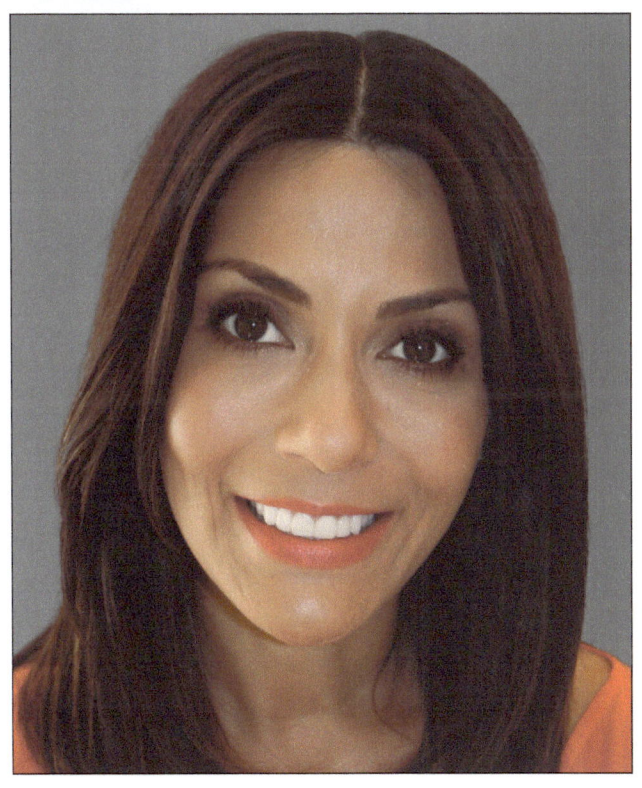

"The patient came by and I saw I could do a few things rather easily to greatly enhance her smile. I went back to my friend at that point to say I was in, and that show ended up being the first in a long line of them. One show seemed to lead to another one.

"Though there were several, and they were all interesting in their own way, there are two that really stick out in my memory. The first one was an incredible story covered on the first makeover show out of Europe, which was called Extreme Makeover London.

"The person we were doing a makeover on for this show was a teacher out of England who had Multiple Sclerosis, which is a condition that creates a lot of muscular pain and the vertebra starts to change shape, putting a lot of pressure on the body.

"She was going to be here in Beverly Hills for 6 weeks getting all kinds of work done including a facelift, an eyebrow lift, a nose job, Lasik, and I was doing the teeth. It was going to be a complete transformation. And the whole makeover was going to start with my segment.

"What really made this case interesting was not the amount of work being done, but the fact that she was in pain all of the time. She couldn't really sit for too long.

"Also, a lot of people don't really know this, but on these makeover shows the patients are getting put to sleep a lot to get the work done, and one of the side effects of general anesthesia can be temporary depression.

"If you're just put under one time this won't really happen, but if you're put under several times in a very short period like that, it's something I've seen happen time and time again.

"I was concerned about this with her. She was here all by herself so far away from home, and she had this added element of pain. It was a lot to deal with, so I would sit with her for hours and just talk to her to make sure that she was doing okay. I also decided that I didn't want to put her under myself, even though I usually would have for the amount of work we were going to be doing.

"During one of these conversations I asked her who knew she was doing all of this, and she told me that no one did. As far as anyone at home knew she was on a sabbatical.

"I asked her what she thought everyone's reaction was going to be. She said she really didn't know what people were going to think. This kind of work was very unusual where she was from at the time.

"I got this feeling at that point that this was not going to go over very well, and I told her that. I knew the mentality at the time in that part of the world was that if you're doing something to change the way you look then there was something psychologically wrong with you. I really didn't think they would go for it.

"It took a very long time to get the work done because she was in so much pain that we had to take a lot of breaks. I even had someone there to massage her back to help her tolerate being in the chair for that long, but it was very difficult for her.

"Nevertheless, this case turned out beautifully. It was the greatest transformation I have ever been a part of because there were so many different, incredibly talented people that were involved.

"It was so satisfying to see someone who never thought that she was going to be pretty enough to even get asked out on a date, suddenly have really high hopes in just 6 weeks."

"That's really cute."

"It was, and she was a very nice person that we all sort of fell in love with, so it was really heart-warming to see it happen and to be a part of it.

"However, that's not where it ended because then she went back for the reveal, and immediately people started to attack her for what she had done."

"You're kidding me. Did she look completely different?"

"She looked great. That transformation was done by such skilled experts that all the work looked very natural. If you hadn't known her before you might not have ever known she had anything done at all.

"She went on many different talk shows and radio shows to talk about the transformation since this was such a new idea, and as I had feared, it was not received well. People would call in and say, 'What's wrong with you? You're crazy.' She was told she should go see a psychiatrist. It was really out of hand."

"That seems terrible. How did she feel about it?" I asked.

"She told me if she could go back in time and do it over knowing what she knows, she would do it all again because what she had gained in quality of life and how she now felt about herself was so much more than what anyone could say to her. It really didn't matter.

"Then a year went by, and she was actually laid off from her teaching job because it had become such a circus. There were people waiting outside the school to take photos of her, and she was being slandered in the newspapers. It was a complete overreaction, and I'm sure it was hard on her to some degree, but the story actually has a happy ending."

"Oh good. I was starting to worry about where this was going."

"I was at the time too, but I knew if she could stay feeling that good about herself and what she had done, that everything would come through in the end. And it really did.

"Five years later all of the initial shock and attacks just sort of disappeared, and things started to change. It turned into this whole movement in England making it okay to improve the way you looked. People were no longer asking her why she had done it, but asking her for advice on what could be done. She was finally able to share her story the right way."

"Did you keep in touch with her?"

"Absolutely. She comes by every year or so for me to check her teeth and say hello, and she's doing really well.

"It was one of those situations where no one ever could have guessed what they were getting into from the beginning, and there were so many ups and downs, but in the end it really is a happy story. Which is why it really stuck in my mind."

"What's the other case? You mentioned there were two."

"All of the work that I did on the show Ten Years Younger. That show was exceptional for a few reasons.

"Firstly, I was working with a number of other experts to get everything done on someone in only 10 days. That would have been hard enough, but in actuality it was even worse because *I* only had one day with the camera crew in my office to get whatever my portion of the work was done.

"It was one thing if it was just some whitening or something like that, but if we had to make veneers or crowns, it was a whole other story.

"There's no possible way to get veneers and crowns in just a few hours, because you have to send the molds to the lab, which meant that the temporaries that I put on people had to be so good that no one would know they were just temporaries.

"They had to be that convincing because the week after, when that person would go into the studio to talk about everything, he or she would have the real thing on, and it would have to match. The temporaries had to be perfect.

"I was on that show for 4 seasons, on over a dozen episodes, and as time went on…"

"You got really good at temporaries." I interjected, laughing.

"You do get really good at temporaries, and you know what else you get good at? You get really good at predicting what problems you're going to run into between where you are and where you're going to end up, which also makes you really good at solving those things on the spot and resolving them in such a way that someone watching would never know you were having a hard time with anything."

"How long would you actually have?"

"About 3 hours to do all the work."

"Oh wow. That sounds extremely stressful."

"It is. Having a week to work on something suddenly seemed like a luxury. And the interesting thing was that in the beginning the show worked with multiple dentists, but as the seasons went by, they started to narrow down until I was really the only one doing it."

This was no surprise to me at all. "They must have loved you," I said, and he nodded.

"The producer came to me and said, 'You're the only one who doesn't complain about this. Everyone else is complaining. You like this, don't you?'

"And he was right. I did. It goes back to that mentality we talked about. I like to be challenged. I like having to figure out how I can do something with what I have in front of me and being able to think on my feet while the camera is on me."

"Of course you love that."

"It is the key to being able to do well in this field."

"You have to get a little nervous in situations like that."

"Of course I do. People ask me that all the time. I do get nervous. I do get worried, but what I do with that feeling is channel it into a solution. I ask myself, what is it that I can do about this? How can I handle it or at least learn something from it so that I can handle it better if the situation ever comes up again?

"I never think, 'I wish I had an easy life.'"

"Yeah, who wants that?" I asked sarcastically, though I do agree with him.

"I actually don't know. I don't know who *would* want a boring life or why they would want a boring life, but a lot of people *do* want that. They want an easy life where they don't have to think.

"There were long periods of time in my practice when I wasn't thinking, and I have to tell you, I was never so miserable. There was nothing to think about. The cases weren't stimulating my mind or making me think on my feet. There's just no way that I would have ever been able to endure that kind of life.

"I know that this is the reason I started to do things the way I do them now, because if you're just doing fillings and crowns and not really changing anything there is nothing to think about. You're pretty much on autopilot, and autopilot to me is like death. I was so bored.

"But when you're going at it from the angle of changing someone's entire face, the width of the arch, the bite, the shape of the teeth, and really the shape of the smile, you really have to think.

"You have to be constantly looking and asking yourself, 'For this particular person how much can I push that lip out? How much can I push the cheek out? How can I get rid of that wrinkle?'

"You have to always be one step ahead of yourself with it. The boredom evaporates. There's no room for boredom when you're dealing with that kind of challenge.

"It's something I have always tried to instill in the people around me. If you don't have that challenge in your life you will lose the zest and passion you have for whatever it is you're doing. Your enthusiasm will wane. That is why I am always looking to do something that will challenge me so that I never lose that passion for this work that I really do love so much.

"It doesn't mean I don't make mistakes. I do. It doesn't mean that there aren't any cases that come up where at some point I'm not happy. It definitely happens. But at the end I'm able to overcome it and get it to a point where I am satisfied, and usually, I have to tell you, if I'm satisfied then the work has far exceeded the patient's wildest dreams for what their smile could look like."

Chapter 3
Clenching and Grinding

82 million Americans have something in common. A nervous habit that plagues twice the number of adults in the country as smoking and is also the number one cause for the most drastic signs of aging that occur in the lower 1/3 of the face. Clenching and grinding wears down teeth, changes the shape of the jaw, causes smile collapse, and most people are not even aware they do it. In this chapter Dr. Maddahi reveals the symptoms of clenching and grinding, how to recognize its effects, and most importantly, how to stop it.

§

Throughout the years, one of the biggest problems I have run into is also one people seem to be the least aware of as a problem, which is the clenching and grinding of teeth. By clenching I mean pressing the teeth tightly against each other, which one might do at night while they sleep or during the day. Clenching is usually caused by stress. By grinding I mean pressing the teeth tightly together and then rubbing the teeth against each other side to side or back and forth. Grinding causes loss of tooth structure, which affects the way someone's upper and lower teeth fit together or their "bite," and is usually caused by the person's bite already being off in some way. We call this a "bad bite," meaning when the upper and lower teeth are closed together there is unevenness in contact throughout the bite, and this unnatural position causes the person who has it to subconsciously try to fix it by grinding the teeth down.

This kind of muscle tension in and around the mouth does more than just affect the teeth; it creates an unnatural squaring of the jaw, thus stripping the natural softness in a face associated with youth.

The person who clenches and grinds will experience the muscles of the jaw line and cheeks bulking out with overuse, giving the lower 1/3 of the face a boxy shape. If you clench your teeth together very tightly and look in a mirror you will see the muscles protruding out, which can give even the most feminine woman a masculine look.

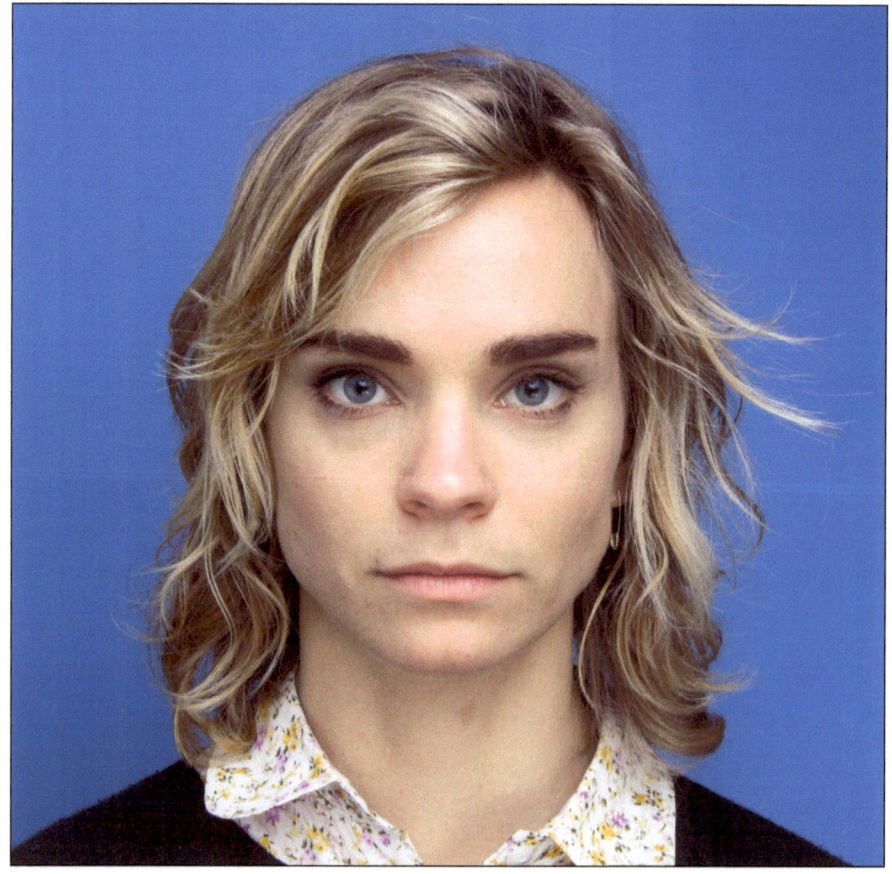

Clenched Jaw

When a patient sits down in my chair for the first time, I can immediately tell if they clench because of the way their jaw muscles look. On the outside there are protruding muscles on either side of the jaw, and on the inside, if they are grinding, there will be wear marks on the teeth. Severe grinding will cause teeth to be worn down to such an extent that the bite will over-close, causing the chin to jut forward and deep lines to develop in the corners of the lips.

Grinding will also make the front teeth appear too short and uneven.

Teeth being worn down, jaw lines being boxy, and the chin jutting forward are all things that add years to someone's face and are *all* as

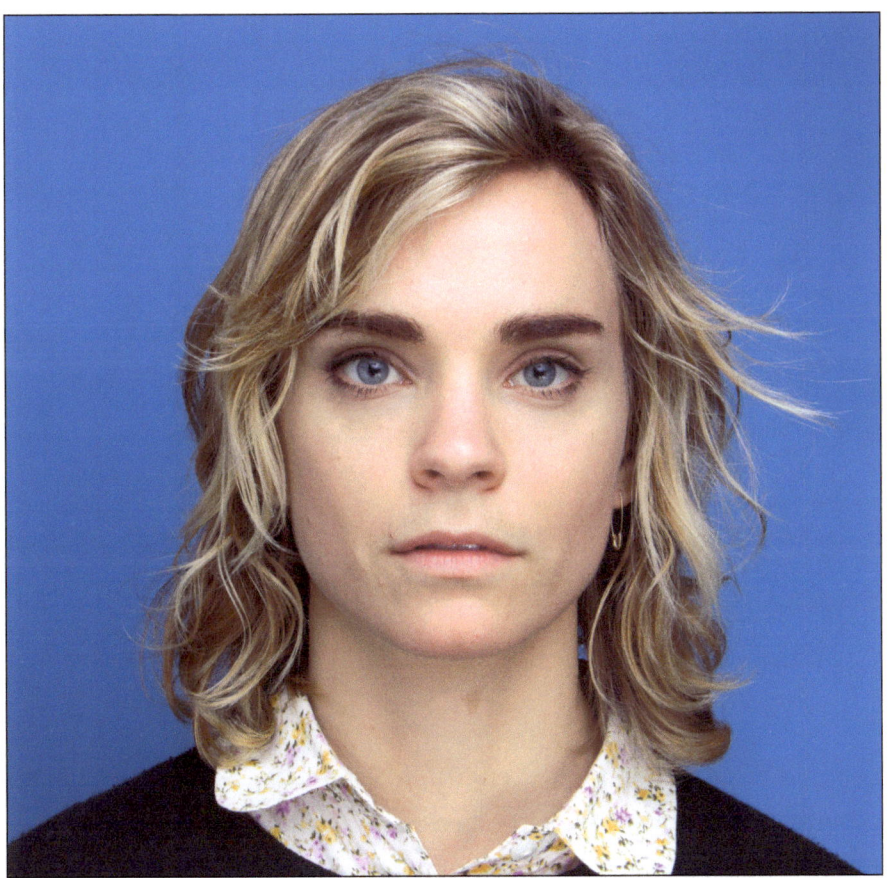

Unclenched Jaw

a result of clenching and grinding of the teeth. In dentistry the main remedy for clenching and grinding is to make someone a night guard to wear while they sleep.

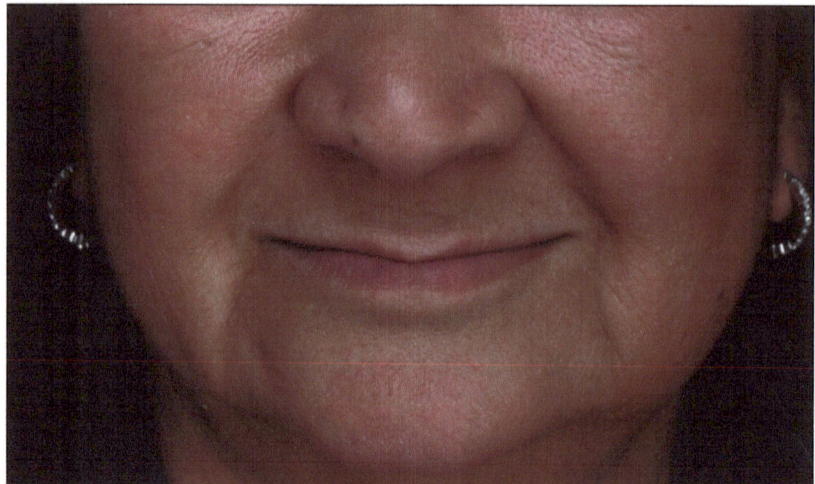

Collapsed Jaw Before

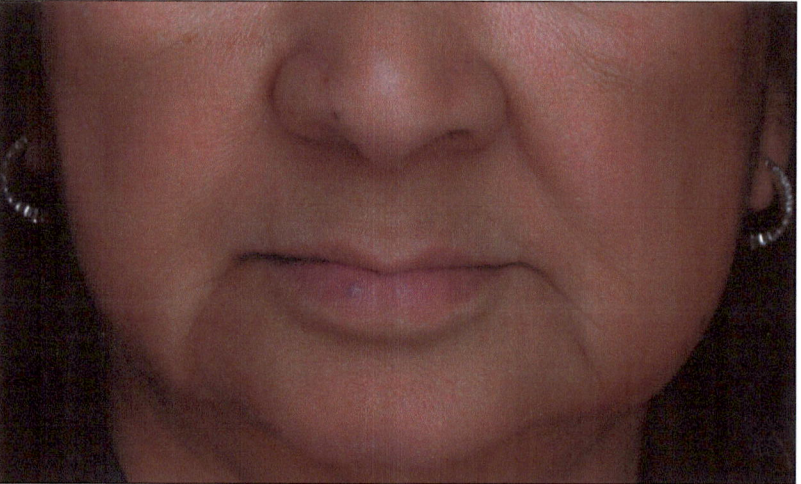

Collapsed Jaw After

This night guard does three things. Firstly, because it is one piece of hard plastic it dissipates the pressure on any one particular tooth in the mouth, making it impossible to put any pressure on individual teeth. This will, over time, relax the muscles and stop them from bulging out. It will also stop or greatly reduce headaches and jaw aches in the morning, which are caused by this tension in the muscles. The next thing the guard does is stop one from wearing down the teeth, as they are protected with the plastic. The last and most important thing is the protection of the tendon that sits in between the jawbone and the socket. This tendon, like any other tendon, is susceptible to irreversible damage if worn down. You see this in athletes with worn down tendons in their knees, elbows, or shoulders. Eventually as the tendon wears down, there will be bone on bone contact which produces a lot of pain, and there is no real solution to completely reverse the damage done. This is the most important function of the night guard.

A night guard is a great non-invasive remedy for someone who is clenching and/or grinding at night (which is most common). However, I have come across many patients that are exhibiting this nervous habit during the day. There are even some cases where the bulking of the muscles in the jaw are due to that person's diet. This is found in someone who eats a lot of crunchy food, such as almonds and granola, or someone who chews a lot of gum.

One of the most difficult things about treating clenching and grinding is that most people are not aware of it. I had to come up with a question that would make someone aware of his or her own clenching and grinding. I tried many different questions over the years until I finally landed on this one: "Do you ever feel your teeth touching during the day?"

If the answer to this question is yes, then I know this person is clenching and/or grinding. In a resting position your teeth should not be touching. Even when you eat, your teeth should not touch, and someone who has this habit has to be made aware that this is unnatural in order to fix it.

Anti-Aging Dentistry

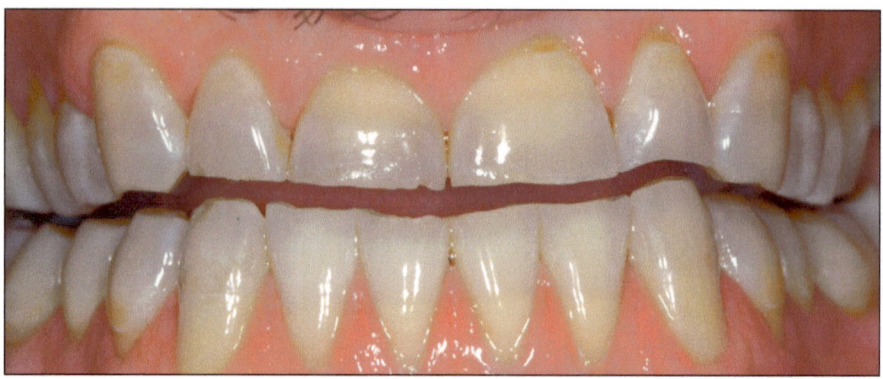

Front Teeth Uneven & Worn Before

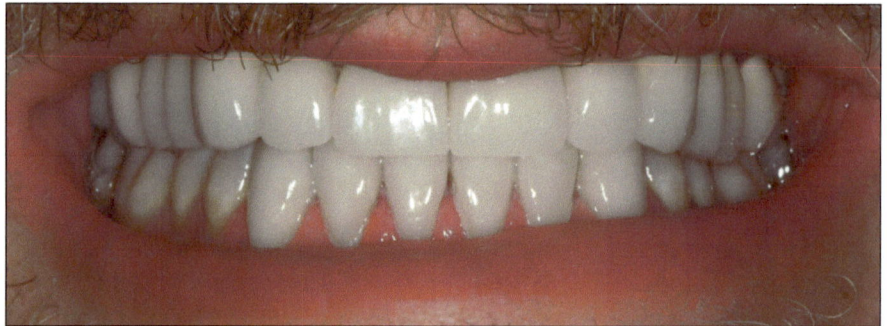

Front Teeth Uneven & Worn After

Normally when asked this question the patient will come back in a week or so shocked at how much they've noticed they do clench or grind their teeth. They'll tell me they've found themselves doing it while they're in the car, or lifting weights, or when they're concentrating on a computer, and in some cases just this level of awareness can be enough to stop it. Of course, I can provide someone with a guard to wear when they do certain activities, but mostly I just recommend being cognizant of the problem and the damage it's doing and the patient will correct it on their own.

The other problem that comes up with clenching and grinding is how much time it adds to the bite adjustment phase of Anti-Aging Dentistry procedures. In severe cases it can take more than double the amount of time it normally takes, anywhere from 2 weeks to several months, before everything is comfortable and perfect.

This is due to the fact that when someone has been clenching and grinding they have stretched the ligaments around the jaw joint. This allows the jaw to move around in many additional directions than is normal, causing the bite to be constantly changing.

The Symptoms of Clenching

1. Square/boxy jaw line
2. Sensitivity to hot, cold and chewing
3. Jaw ache and headache

The Symptoms of Grinding

1. Square/boxy jaw line
2. Worn down or shorten teeth
3. Collapsed bite
4. Teeth sensitivity to hot cold and/or chewing
5. Jaw ache and or headache

Aging impacts:

1. Lower 1/3 of the face squished
2. Line in the corner of the lips
3. Sagging jaw line

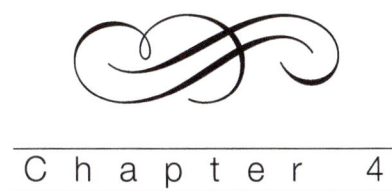

Chapter 4

Food and Habits

The influences of modern day health trends and routines affect everything from the environment we live in to our economy, and they certainly affect the population's health. Dr. Maddahi has compiled here an eye-opening look into how some of these movements have impacted oral health and facial aging.

§

One of the main focuses of my practice has been a kind of preventative dentistry that focuses on bringing awareness to how every day routines might be affecting someone's teeth.

Over the last 27 years I have observed many changes in the problems arising in my patients' mouths. These shifts have invariably coincided with trends in our society's health industry.

As certain foods and diets become popular, there are inevitable evolutions in the symptoms showing up in people's bodies and mouths simultaneously. Everything from a change in gum color to the frequency of broken teeth can be viewed as evidence of a bigger picture shift. I believe in treating the root cause of a problem, as opposed to the symptoms of one, and so it has been important for me to really look at these trends and find alternatives for my patients who follow them.

Cracked Teeth

Over the last decade the number of patients that have come to see me with cracked or broken teeth has risen. As with any increase that's fairly sudden like this, I immediately become wary of an underlying movement.

When teeth are broken or cracked it is usually as a result of clenching and grinding, and some of my colleagues were quick to blame an increase in stress equaling an increase in this habit. That is a logical explanation to a certain point, but it wouldn't explain an increase of this size, so I began to ask my patients questions about their eating habits to see if anything made sense.

What I found was a pattern that came from the question, "What is the hardest food you eat?" I noticed that often the answer would be whole almonds, which have become popular in recent years due to several reports on their health benefits.

One patient specifically worked as a sort of guinea pig to help prove this theory. He was a young man who came in to see me because he was experiencing an extreme amount of pain while chewing, as well as sensitivity to hot and cold. This kind of pain in the mouth is typically due to decay, infection and root exposure, or years of constant pressure on the teeth associated with clenching and grinding.

And yet, this patient had no cavities, infection or root exposure. I thought it had to be clenching and grinding, but upon further inspection it became clear that he didn't do this.

I thought about it awhile before I asked him about his diet. Sure enough he told me he ate a lot of nuts, and in particular, a lot of whole almonds.

I decided to try an experiment. I asked him to simply give up the almonds for one week. When he came back to see me 7 days later, he reported that 50% of the pain was completely gone. I told him to go one more week, in which time he also gave up all other nuts, and sure enough, before he knew it, all the pain had vanished.

It's important to note here that I agree with the health benefits of almonds and do not want to stop people from eating them, which is why the experiment didn't end there.

I decided to find an alternative that would allow my patients to still eat nuts without having to damage their teeth or experience this kind of sensitivity. I noticed that what made the almonds so hard to eat was the shape and size of them. To crack a big nut like that someone has to use a lot of torque and it's very hard on the teeth and jaw muscles, which can create a lot of sensitivity over time. The smaller food is between the teeth, the less pressure (thus less torque) is needed to eat it. This was the key to the solution: sliced almonds.

Sliced almonds are still almonds, with all the same health benefits and taste that whole almonds have, but without the shape that makes them so hard on one's teeth.

Stains

Cosmetic Dentistry has been most commonly associated with the whitening of one's teeth. There have been many in-office and at-home remedies for yellowing teeth in the last 10 years, but there are also ways to prevent discoloration and these come from understanding what causes it.

It's generally understood that black teas and coffee stain people's teeth. It's also understood that most Americans are not willing to

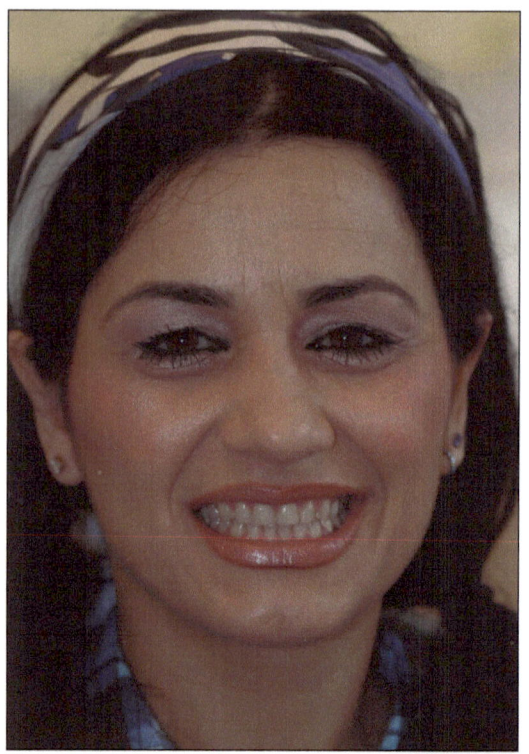

Stained Teeth Before

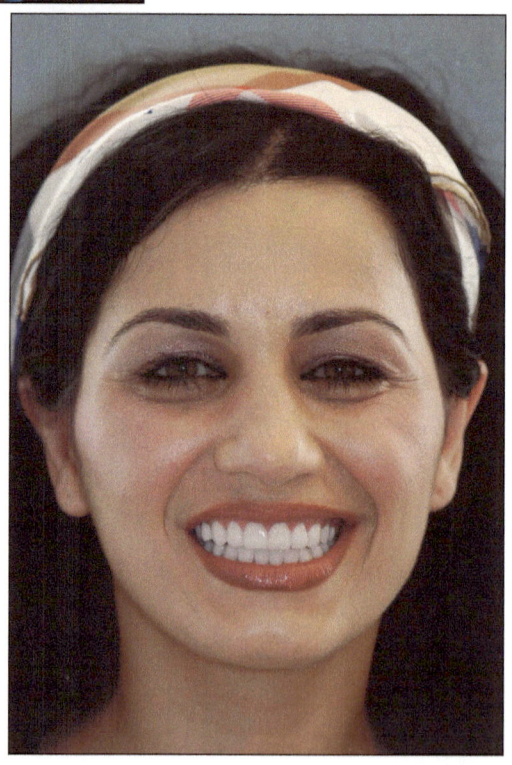

Stained Teeth After

give caffeine up. So, the question has become, "How can people drink coffee and/or tea without staining their teeth?" Not, "How can I get people to stop drinking it?"

The answer to this riddle came from fashion models, actually. I have worked on many models over the years and have noticed a very unique staining pattern on their teeth. They have a lot of stains on the back of their teeth and none on the front. I asked a few of them how many cups of coffee they were drinking a day and was astonished to learn that, because these women work 12 to 14 hour days, they drink endless cups of coffee to keep them awake.

It seemed impossible that their teeth would be so white if that were the case, and when I said so I found out something interesting. They all used an industry secret when drinking coffee, a straw. Drinking their coffee through a straw was keeping their teeth white and allowing them to drink as much as they want.

Straws to drink staining liquid through has been the solution I have given my patients for years now, and this trick has helped them avoid a lot of discoloration. Straws and vented lids (like the ones you get on your hot drinks from Starbucks) work because they bring the liquid back behind your teeth.

It has been especially helpful in the prevention of grey stains on teeth that have shown up more and more with the growing popularity of green tea.

The benefits of green tea became wide-spread knowledge some years ago, and the traditional Asian drink has become widely accepted as a healthier alternative to coffee. This is true, and I encourage my patients to drink herbal teas, but the downside to green tea is the stains it leaves behind.

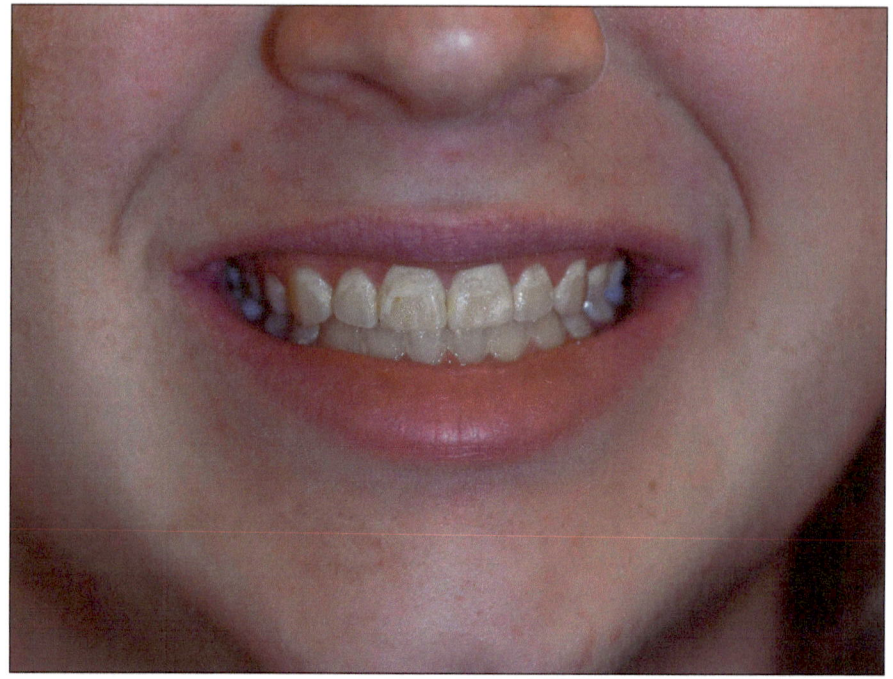

Stained Teeth Before

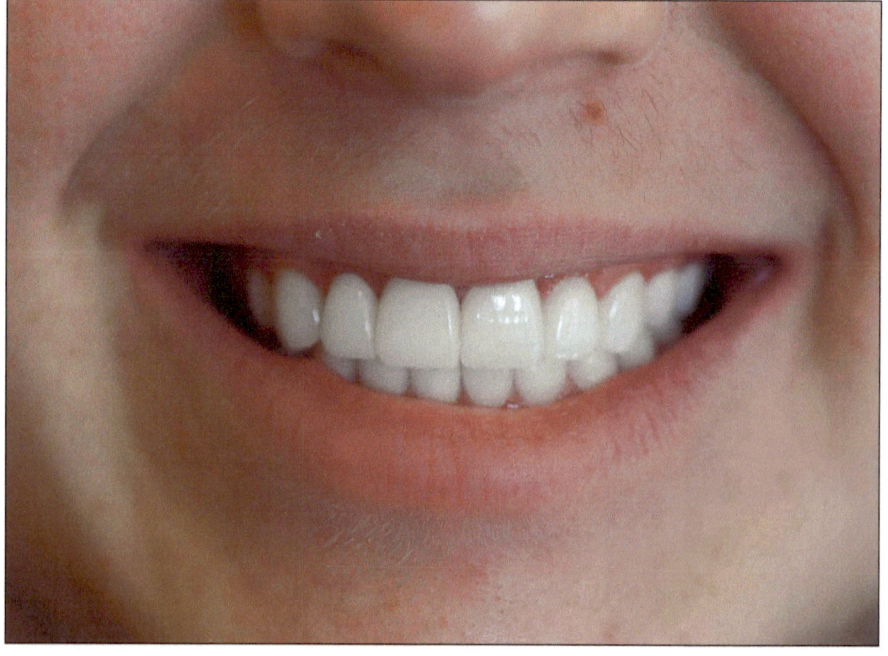

Stained Teeth After

Grey is the hardest color to remove from teeth and is also the most aging color one can have in their mouth. So if someone is going to drink green tea, I highly recommend they drink it out of a straw, or ideally, a vented lid, as these lids require less pursing of the lips, which is an action that can create wrinkles similar to the ones smokers develop over time.

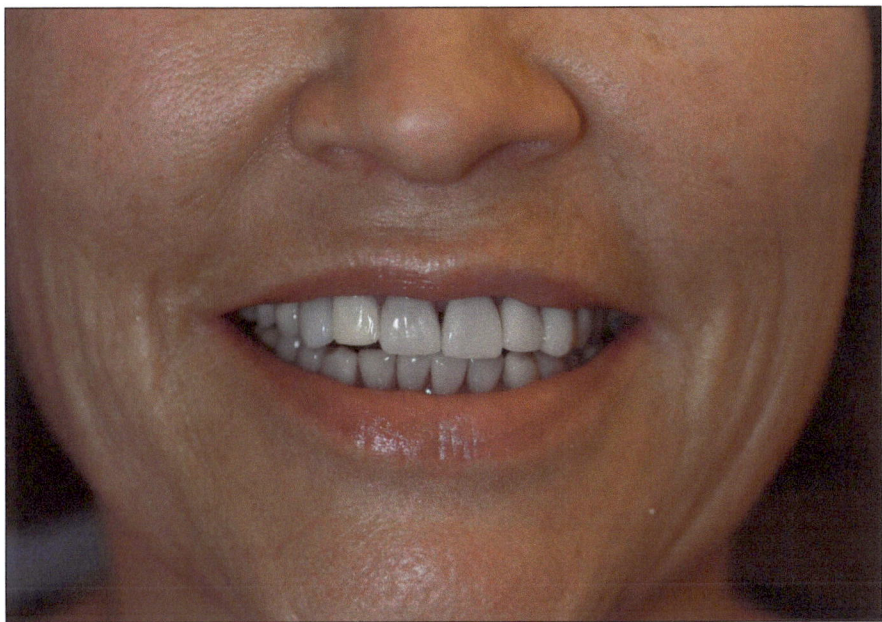

Grey Stains

Right around when green tea became popular, there was another push in the health industry, and that was the push for antioxidants focused mainly around blueberries. Antioxidants have several amazing health benefits and even have anti-aging properties, but much like green tea, blueberries (and other dark berries) leave grey stains on people's teeth. The best way to get the benefits of these antioxidant and vitamin rich fruits without incurring the stains they leave is to drink them in a smoothie with a straw.

The last item I'd like to touch on is also the one I can't say I have a good solution for yet, which is red wine. There are many perks to drinking a glass of red wine, so the fact that it stains teeth worse than just about anything else poses a problem. I can hardly tell my patients to drink it through a straw.

The only way I've been able to lessen the stains drinking red wine causes is by having my patients brush their teeth as soon as they're done drinking it. This does seem to help quite a bit. The patient is removing the wine from the surface of the tooth before it sets in and leaves much of a stain. And since most people drink red wine at home to unwind, it's not a terribly inconvenient thing to do either.

Gum Health

There is no substitute for a consistent regimen of flossing when it comes to taking care of your gums, and getting patients to do this has its challenges, but there is one trend that I noticed also gave a considerable boost to the health of people's gums in recent years.

Some time ago I began to notice an upsurge in the healthy pink that we, as dentists, look for in our patients' gums. The strange thing was that the patients I was seeing this shift in really didn't have the best oral hygiene. It was very puzzling.

In dental school you learn that there are two different kinds of bacteria that can be found in someone's mouth. There's the kind that makes you prone to cavities and the kind that makes you prone to gum disease.

At first, it would have been easy to just assume that the people I was seeing with these very pink gums were lacking the bacteria that causes gum inflammation, ultimately making someone gum disease-proof, but after awhile there just seemed to be too many of these cases for that to be the reason.

Restoring Youth, One Smile at a Time

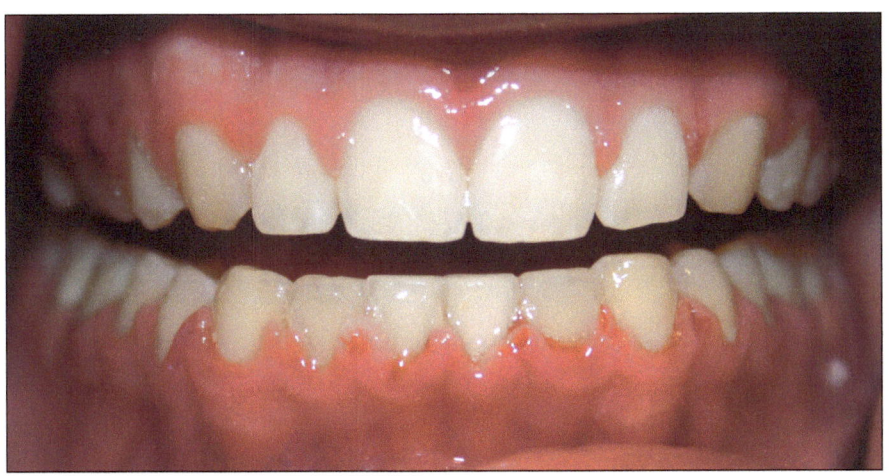

Unhealthy Gums

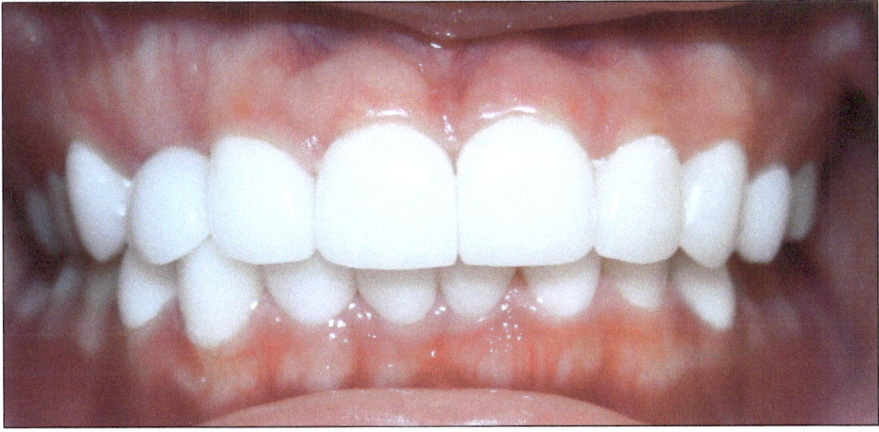

Healthy Gums

I started to think about this and what could possibly be creating that kind of change. One day the answer came to me when I was seeing a patient of mine who was pregnant.

When women are experiencing a sudden excess of hormones, like they do when they're pregnant, their gums bleed more.

This got me thinking about the flip side. If extra hormones created more bleeding in someone's gums, then it would stand to reason that fewer hormones would mean less bleeding.

I started to ask my patients who came in with these healthy looking gums if they ate organic food or inorganic food, and one for one the answer came back "mostly organic." These people were experiencing a healthier gum because what they were eating was missing the kinds of hormones that are found in inorganic foods.

It's a pretty interesting upshot to eating organic, but it is also a reflection of a bigger picture in whole body health. If that's the effect hormones in the food we eat are creating on our gums, I'm completely certain there are other consequences going on in the rest of our bodies.

Wear and Tear

On top of all the foods we eat that may do damage to our teeth, shift our bite, or cause unnatural wrinkles over time, there are also habits that we may have no idea are affecting our faces.

The first example of this I'd like to point out is a slight unevenness in the wrinkles of someone's face I will often times see. They may have a deeper line on one side of their mouth than the other, and when I ask them which side they sleep on the answer is always the side that has the deeper line.

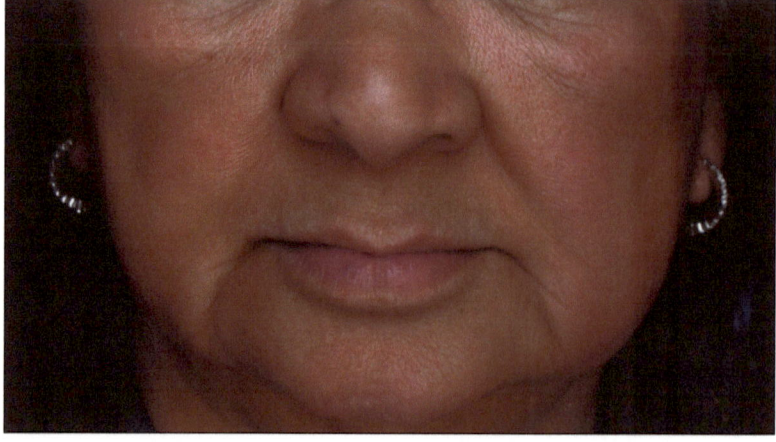

Wrinkles Deeper on One Side Than the Other

These kinds of changes can typically be explained, and because I am approaching dentistry from an Anti-Aging angle I am always looking for the patterns, because that's where the solutions lie.

Another example like this is the wrinkles that form around someone's lips that I have mentioned, which are usually associated with smoking.

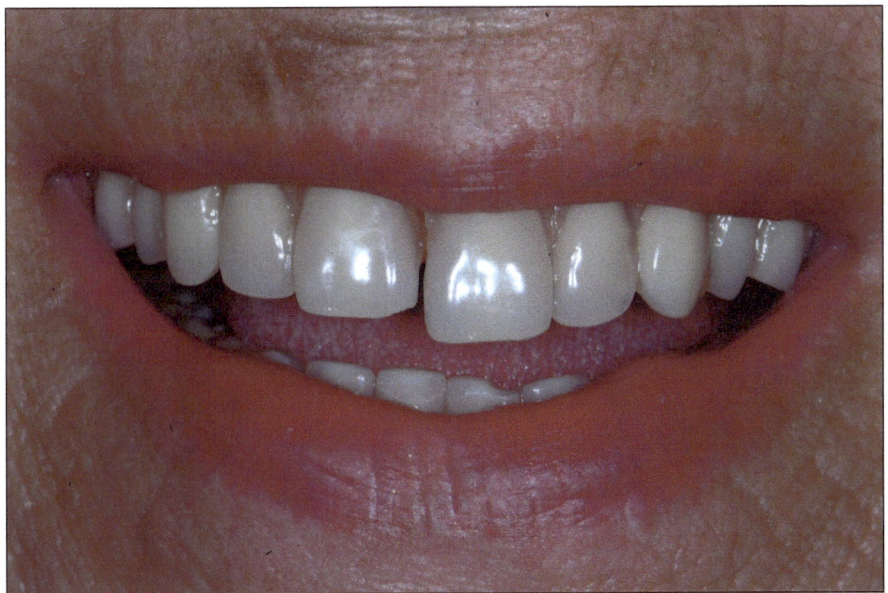

Wrinkles Around the Lips

I have found, however, that these wrinkles occur in many people who do not smoke. They can form from the overuse of straws, and I have even seen patients who display the pursed lips that create these lines only when they are concentrating.

Years of this can result in wrinkles, and these particular wrinkles are the hardest to get rid of, so when I start to see them appearing in my patients I am quick to draw attention to whatever area in their life this habit exists.

There are some routines that can be found in people's workday that could be doing quite a bit of damage as well. There have been patients who have come in to see me who exhibit signs of clenching and grinding, but they do not clench and grind. To figure out what could be causing this I had to ask a lot of questions and look at it from a number of angles. Finally I came up with some pretty interesting answers.

The first one has to do with those of my patients who have office jobs. A lot of people who sit at a desk for 8 hours may spend a lot of that time looking down to read. If you try this you can feel that you are actually pushing your lower jaw into your top jaw. Hours of this, day after day, can result in neck and jaw aches.

Similarly, when people sit with their chin in the palm of their hand they're pushing their upper and lower jaw together. This kind of pressure may seem harmless, but if it is a part of someone's constant routine it can create pressure on the upper jaw much like the kind one would find in someone who was clenching.

Through all my years of paying attention to my patients' faces and what changes in them over time, the thing I've always known is there is an answer to everything that happens to us as we begin to look older. If I can find the answer I can also find the solution, and this way of thinking has been what's made Anti-Aging Dentistry possible.

Chapter 5

Support From Inside

The appearance of wrinkles and lines in one's face as they age comes from one simple thing, the waning of support. All manner of cosmetic procedures have been developed to correct this and reverse it, but there are those that have remained a mystery or have proved difficult to improve. The procedures of Anti-Aging Dentistry have handled some of these key aging issues and greatly lessened the need for fillers and the invasive procedures of plastic surgery.

§

One of the wrinkles that appears over time that puzzles my patients the most is the deep horizontal line that I've mentioned in one or both corners of the mouth.

This line, up until now, has been widely regarded as impossible to fix. It is also a perfect example of what Anti-Aging Dentistry is able to provide in comparison with other cosmetic procedures. I have talked to many Dermatologists who have all said the same thing, which is that no matter how many fillers someone gets in the area surrounding the mouth this particular line is just not going to go away. It's been a bit of a mystery.

Over the years as I developed some of these procedures, I have been able to solve this mystery and make this line significantly less

Anti-Aging Dentistry

visible by building up the teeth, which provides the vertical support that's missing from inside the mouth.

This line only appears because the bite is collapsed, meaning it's too far closed, and this puts a constant amount of pressure on the mouth by squishing the lips.

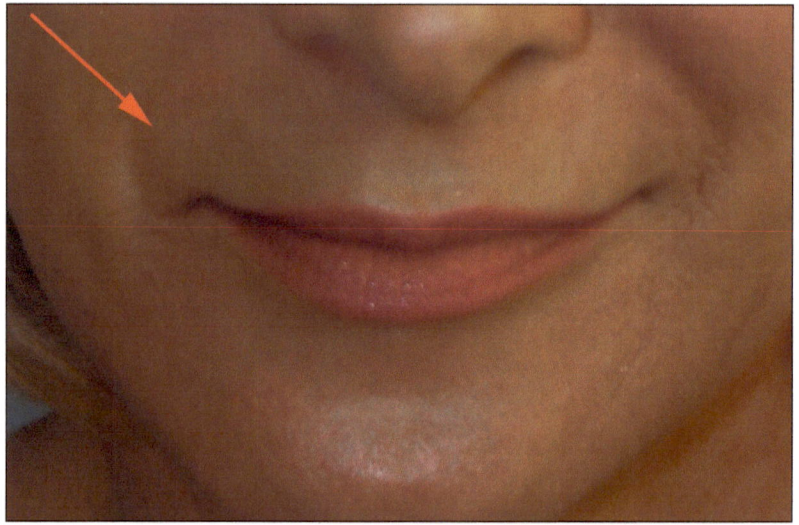

Deep Lines in the Corners of the Mouth Before

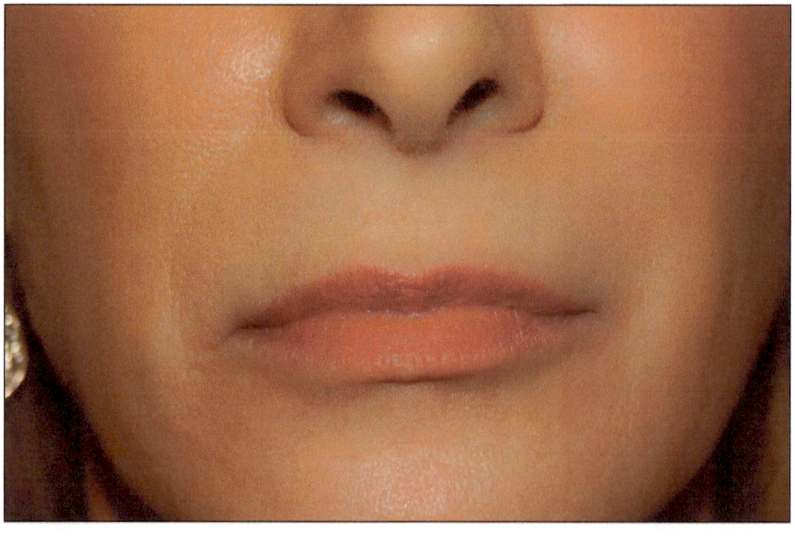

Deep Lines in the Corners of the Mouth After Procedure

This concept of adding more tooth structure with porcelain veneers and crowns, thus providing permanent support where there isn't any, is the one that changed the game and transformed Cosmetic Dentistry into Anti-Aging Dentistry. The idea is that a lot of wrinkles and lines that appear around the mouth over time cannot be wholly fixed with fillers. A filler may provide some temporary decrease in their visibility, but cannot erase them totally, and they will continue to resurface and get worse without proper support.

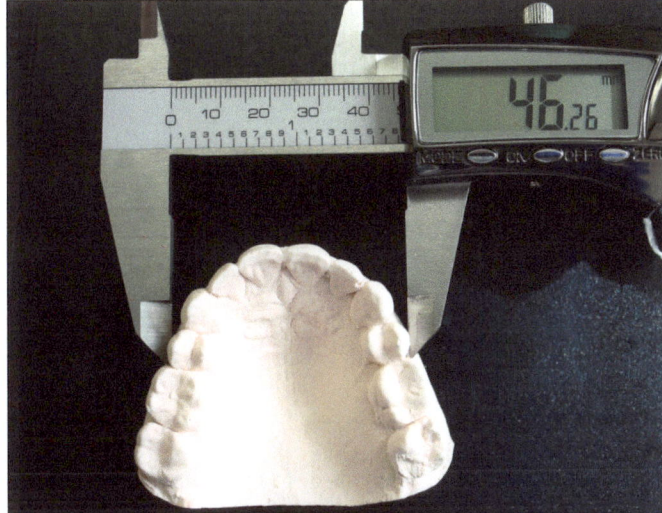

Mold of Upper Teeth Before

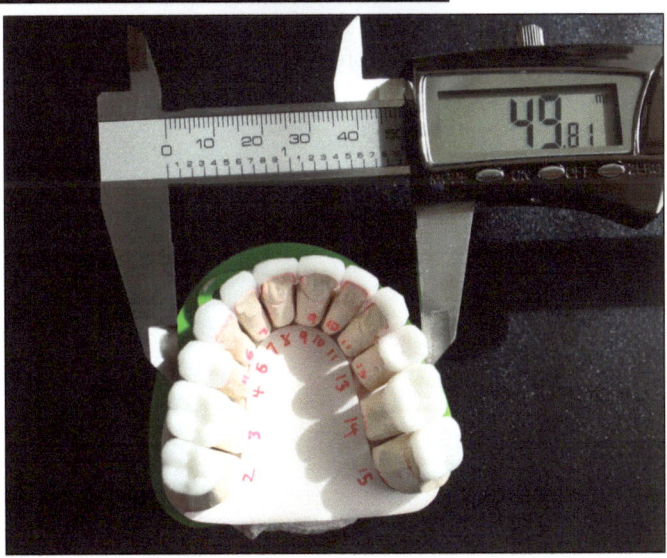

Mold of Upper Teeth After

Although this horizontal line only becomes acutely apparent in later years due to chronic compression from the bite being too closed, causing the corners of the mouth to constantly be creasing, the truth is that if one had enough vertical support from the teeth these lines would not appear in the first place.

The only long-term solution to fix this line is to open up the bite enough that the face is no longer squished. And the only way to open up the bite is with Anti-Aging Dentistry by providing extra length to the teeth, thus creating space where it had been missing. However, there are dangers in opening the bite too much as well; firstly, the teeth may look too long which reduces the esthetics of the smile and secondly, if the teeth become too long it can create difficulty pronouncing letters such as "S" or "Z" or "Ch".

Opening up the bite the proper amount will do two major things. It will make this horizontal line decrease considerably, and it will uncompress the lower 1/3 of the face, which is the most drastic change someone will see from these procedures. This lengthening softens the patient's face so much that it will appear as if they have had much more than just their teeth done.

Opening the bite by making teeth longer has the following effects on the face:

- Lifts the lower 1/3 of the face

- Gets rid of or greatly reduces the horizontal line on the corner of the lips

- Helps with sagging jaw line

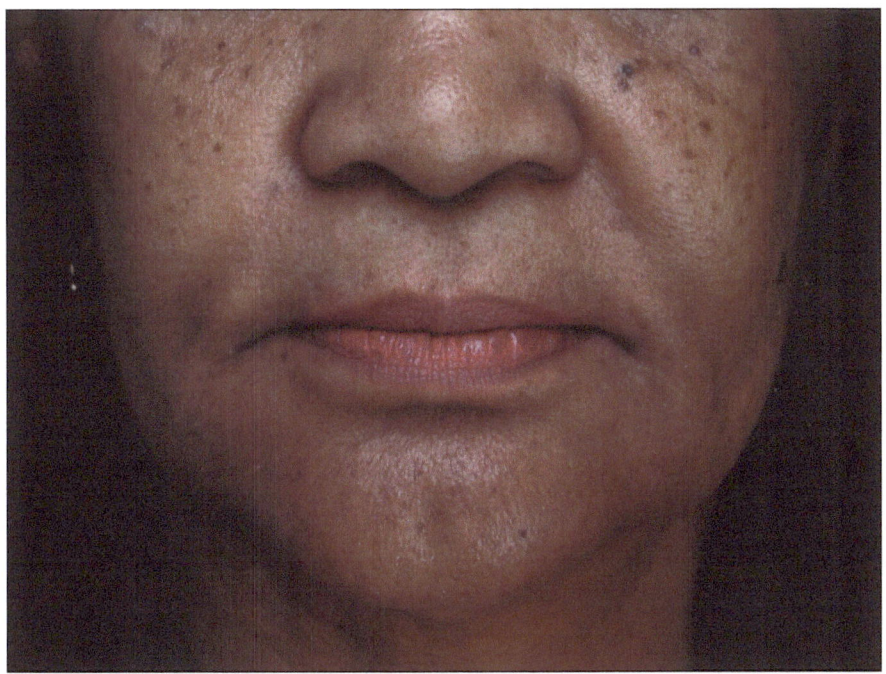

Squished Lower 1/3 of the Face

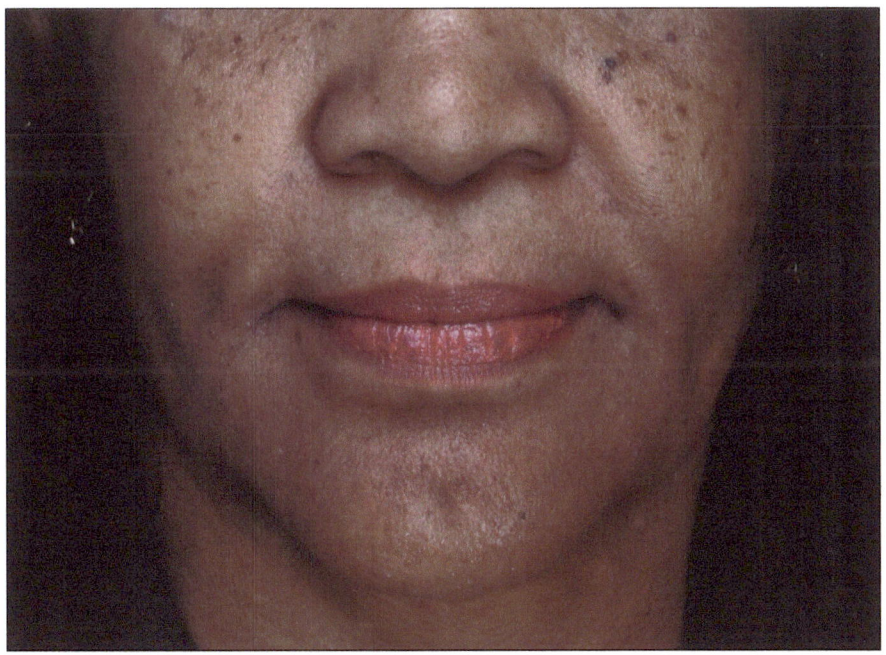

Squished Lower 1/3 of the Face After

Lip Support

Building out the teeth so that they're thicker than they were has a different set of benefits. It gives someone fuller lips and plumps the cheeks by widening the arch or providing better lip support.

In this photo, you can see the top lip comes out from the base of the nose at an angle. This changes as one ages and the fatty tissue within the lip gradually disappears. When teeth are tilted inward and not in the proper position to support the lip, it will begin to roll under as the youthful plump starts to vanish. If the teeth are supporting the lip it cannot curl in as much, so the lip will appear fuller than it would have.

Tilted teeth are largely due to genetics and can only be corrected with veneers or braces. There are drawbacks and benefits to both solutions. Braces can be utilized very successfully to both straighten teeth and to bring them out for support. Unfortunately, the success of braces in providing support is greatly decreased as someone gets older. Once the bone has fully formed around age 16, braces can no longer be used to widen someone's arch, and if they are used to bring out tilted-in teeth there will inevitably be spaces between them.

If one opts for veneers and crowns they will not have to worry about spaces, and the arch can be widened, but it must also be understood that getting them put on requires a loss of tooth structure, and though the technological advancements are making it possible for patients to keep their veneers longer than ever, they still need to be replaced every so often.

However, the benefits to adding porcelain veneers to one's teeth for Anti-Aging purposes are very clear and are the reasons these procedures have been called facelift alternatives. The patient will have a fuller, more vibrant look that will last much longer than any filler on the market and the results will look much more natural.

Restoring Youth, One Smile at a Time

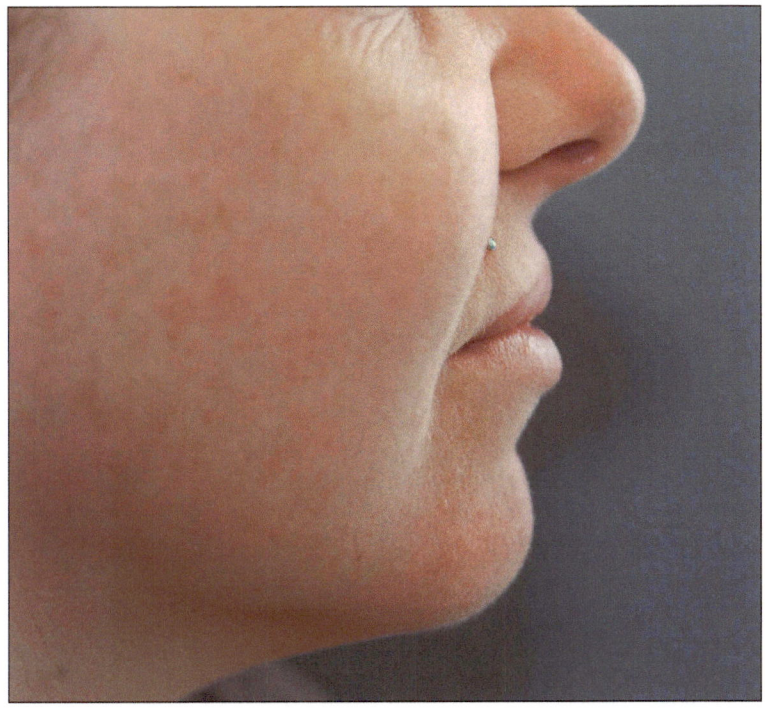

Unsupported Lips

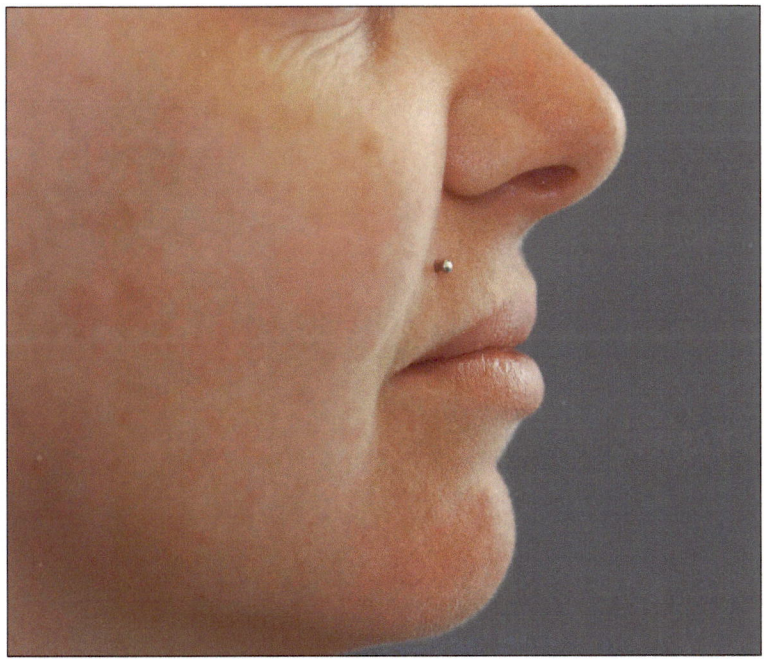

Supported Lips

Benefits of building out front teeth:

1. Decrease wrinkles on upper lip
2. Make the upper lip plumper

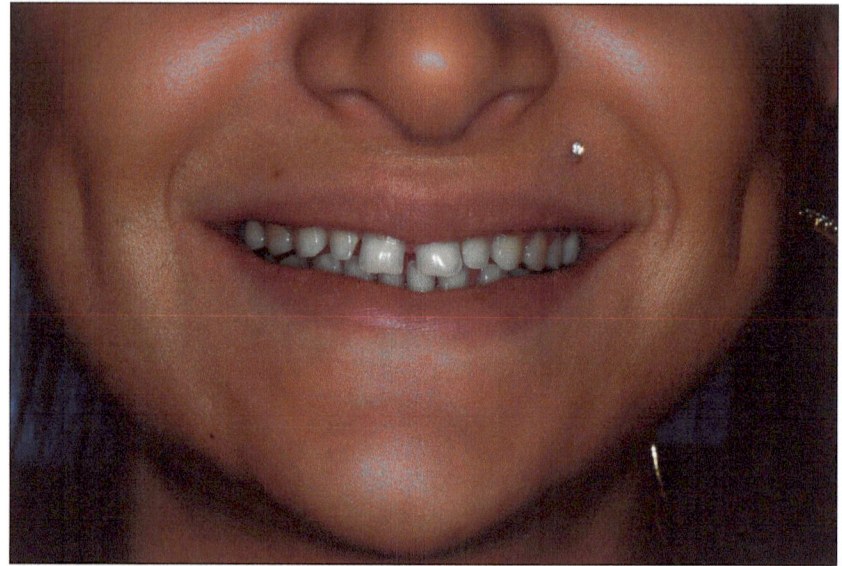

Teeth with Spaces Before

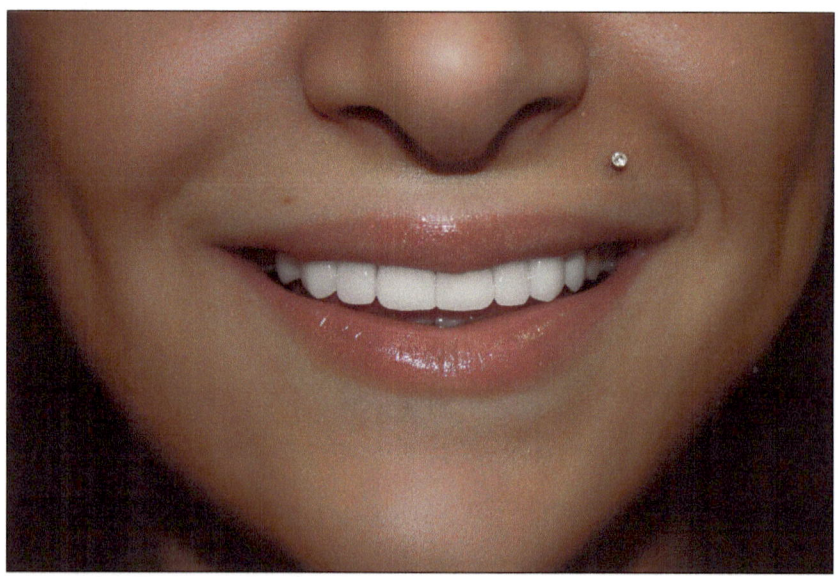

Teeth with Spaces After

Widening The Arch

There is one thing that every iconic smile has in common.

When looking at a smile like this one it is easy to see the beauty in it, but understanding *what* makes it beautiful is the only way to recreate it. I have spent many hours dissecting popular smiles to figure out why they are.

The first thing I see in Halle Berry's smile is the fullness of it. Her smile is wide, and all you see is straight, white teeth in it. There are no spaces or black holes. This is because she has the proper arch form, meaning the arch of her teeth is wide enough that it fills up the mouth.

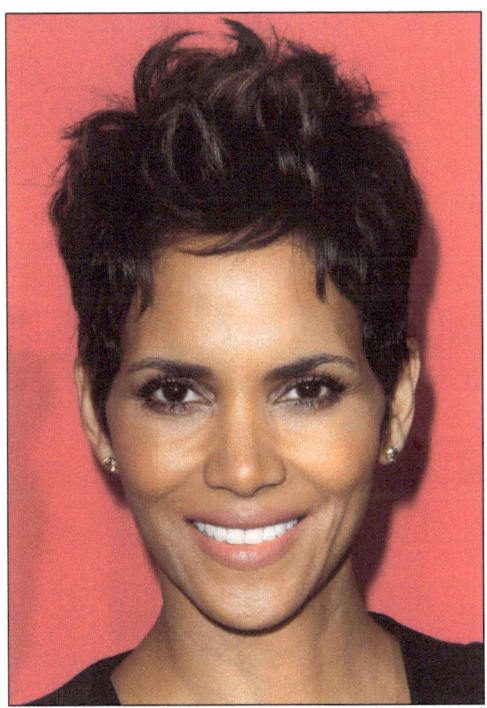

Actress Halle Berry

This is the number one thing that separates a beautiful, aesthetic smile from one that is less so.

Anti-Aging Dentistry

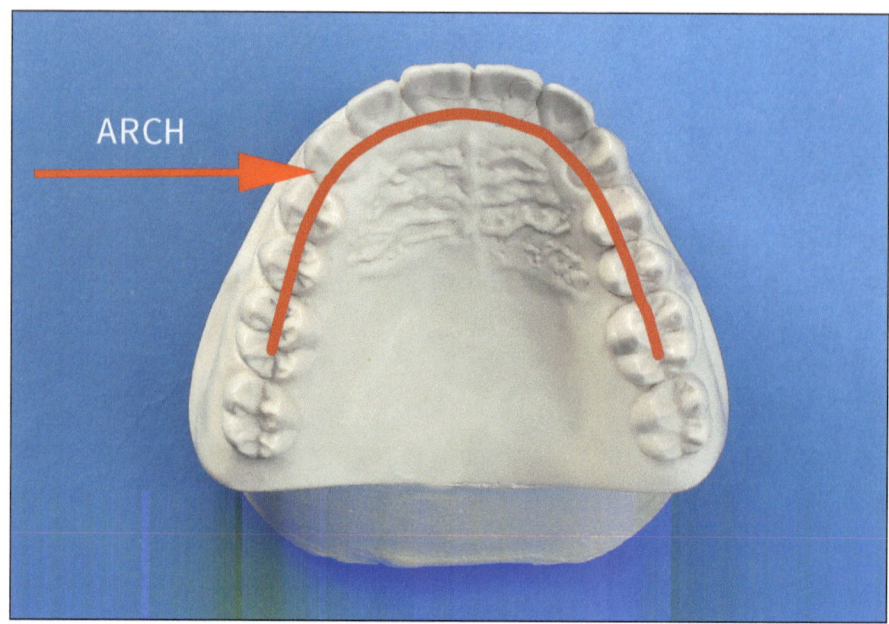

Arch of the Upper Jaw

On the next page you can see black holes that fill up the space between the teeth and the cheeks. These black holes also result in sunken cheeks when someone ages, because of the lack of support from the side teeth.

When the teeth are built out with veneers and crowns, adding width to the arch, these holes are greatly reduced and create the full smile that so many people want. It also provides the added benefit of fuller cheeks, which has a natural lifting effect.

Over the years I have found that the number one reason for a patient having a narrow arch has been the removal of the 4 bicuspid teeth (side teeth next to the eye teeth) due to over crowding (teeth being crooked due to lack of space) by Orthodontists. In recent years this practice has lessened and has been replaced by widening the arch instead of teeth extractions.

Benefits of widening the arch:

1. Wider and fuller smile line

2. Decreased black holes on the side of the cheeks while smiling

3. Provides cheek support

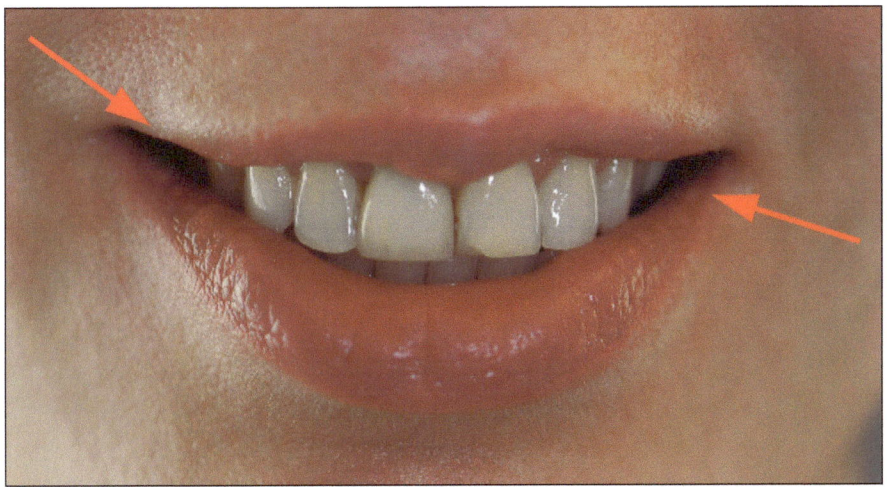

Smile with Black Holes

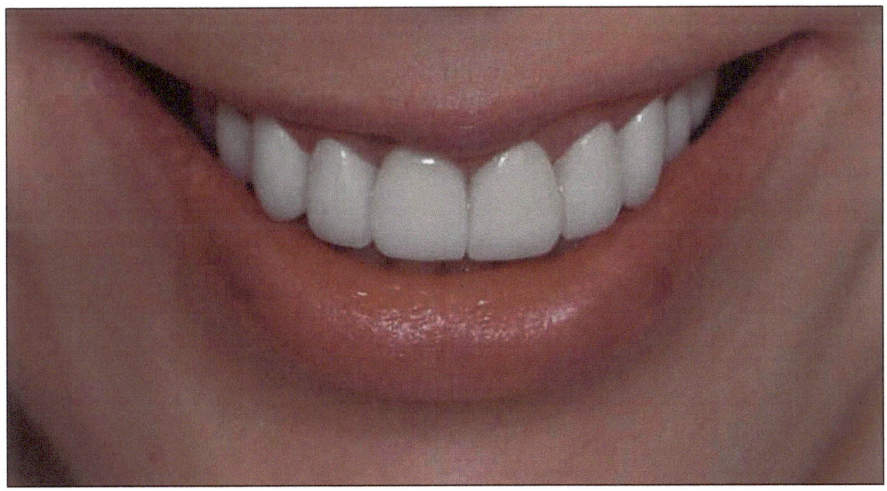

Smile without Black Holes

Chapter 6
Technology

To deliver the very best in the medical field you must also operate with the very best in materials and technologies. In this chapter we'll see what cutting edge systems and ideas Dr. Maddahi has in place in his offices to deliver the fastest and best results the industry has to offer.

§

I have always focused a lot of energy on being as ahead of the curve as possible in the technology my office uses. It's a huge contributing factor to the speed and efficiency in which I am able to deliver these procedures.

When it comes to technology there is a lot of room for growth in the dental industry. Most practices still use very archaic methods of taking X-Rays, drilling in peoples' mouths, and even the materials that are being used are behind the times.

The first time I really saw this was in regard to X-Rays. About 10 years ago I went on quite a few TV shows to bring awareness to digital X-Rays. Digital X-Rays give you digital images that show up in about 3 seconds on a computer screen. The images are clearer, larger, and can be manipulated so that if they are under or overexposed they don't have to be retaken.

More importantly, you are exposing someone to 90% less radiation, which would be enough all on its own, but there are a couple other key reasons why this is a much better technology.

The materials that are used to develop traditional X-Ray images are biohazardous and to dispose of them safely you have to take a lot of steps, which quite frankly, aren't always taken. With digital X-Rays there are no materials needed to develop the images, making them much safer.

With all of the advantages of digital X-Rays it seemed to me the obvious choice, and so it was shocking to me how difficult it was to get other dentists to make the switch. Many offices still haven't.

The reason for this is the same one many offices still use a lot of out-dated technology, and that is cost and training. These machines cost quite a bit more initially than just sticking to the traditional X-Ray machines they already have. It would also cost quite a bit to train their staff, and on top of that, many dentists still don't have computers in all of their operatories.

So even though they would be saving money in the long run, exposing themselves and their patients to much less radiation and the environment from a lot of biohazardous material, about 50% of the dental industry still use traditional X-Rays.

Advantages of Digital X-Rays

1. Images appear on a computer screen in 3 seconds as opposed to being developed in 5 minutes.

2. Images are clearer and can be enlarged or manipulated if need be.

3. No harmful developmental solutions used, making them environmentally friendly.

4. 90% less radiation for the patient.

Lasers

The next piece of technology that I think is key and is being used even less, is laser technology. Lasers are being used throughout the medical industry to make huge advancements, and yet the dental industry has largely neglected this tool.

I've had my eye on lasers for many years. It took some time before I felt like they were advanced enough to use for my practice, but I truly believe they are the future of the field.

Initially I was just using lasers to detect cavities in my patients, but it wasn't long before I acquired another laser to fix gums by evening them out or lessening the amount that was showing in someone's smile. This was a huge time saver because traditional gum surgery requires 4 to 6 weeks of recovery time before anything further can be done in the mouth.

However, the biggest breakthrough with laser technology in regard to dentistry came with the use of cold lasers. What most people aren't aware of is that the pain in these procedures comes from the heat of the drill coupled with the cold water that is being used to cool the person down. These two things combine to create a lot of sensitivity in the mouth.

One day I was removing a cavity with a cold laser, and I noticed that the cavity was deeper than I had initially thought. Usually I would have to then numb the patient and switch over to a hand drill to continue, and the closer one gets to the nerve the more pain someone is going to experience. This time, however, I did not have to numb the patient. I had the drill at a very slow speed and asked them to tell me if they felt anything, but they did not.

The laser was creating a numbing effect. I began to do further research on this phenomenon and even called the company that produces the lasers, but all the information that was available in regard to this theory was that these lasers seemed to change the chemical structure inside the tooth.

This is what allows me to do a filling over someone's lunch break, and I know, as this technology gets stronger, we'll be using them more and more.

Advantages of Lasers in Dentistry

1. Detect cavities more accurately than with X-Rays

2. In most cases, no need for traditional drills or anesthetics

3. Greatly shortened recovery time, and virtually no post-operation pain.

Hand Drill

The next piece of technology that makes a difference for me is the drill I use. When I first started pushing the boundaries of time in procedures, I noticed that the more I pressed down with my drill the slower it would go.

I realized then that this was because of the airflow that was powering the drill. The more pressure I put on the drill the more the drill would slow down. This made the process of removing metal from the mouth much slower. So I started to look into different kinds of drills that would not be affected by this, which led to my making the switch to an electric hand drill.

It took me quite some time to find one back then, and they are 12 times as expensive as regular hand drills, but it has been a huge time saver for my patients, thus making it a worthwhile investment.

A procedure that might have taken over 6 hours now takes less than 4. This is because the torque stays constant. You're not dealing with the drill slowing down like you would with a regular drill during an increase in pressure.

Another simple discovery was that after a certain point the drill bit (which is called a bur) dulls out, and it starts to take much longer to do any cutting. So I started paying close attention to this and as soon as I felt the slightest indication that the drill was slowing down, I would immediately change out for a new bur.

This has also shaved down the time someone is actually in the chair by quite a bit. It is not cheap to operate this way, because the burs are very expensive, but it takes 20% less time to do this kind of work, so it makes it very worthwhile.

The reason I've focused so much on the speed of my drill is because I have noticed over the years that a huge part of what makes people so uncomfortable with dental procedures is the sound of drilling, so the less I can put someone through that the better.

The Details

There are a few other minutiae that make these procedures so much faster in my office. Everything I do is timed down to the second, so the smallest things need to be whittled down as much as possible.

The first thing we do when we're getting ready to make veneers and crowns for someone is to take a mold of their teeth, so I've made sure I use the fastest setting impression material there is, which means my patients don't have to have their mouths filled up with impression material for very long (usually half the time). I also take two impressions, so that if one of them isn't perfect I have a backup.

Then the impressions go to the lab. I have made sure that everything that's done in my office is done digitally so that things can be accessed immediately. Soon enough this will also be the case with the molds. I don't think we're far off from being able to take 3D digital impressions of a patient's teeth that can be viewed and manipulated on a computer.

To be current one must have computers in all of their operatories and really enjoy technology because it is an ever-evolving game. Every time something new comes out there's a learning curve, and there's always the chance that you'll lose your trained staff and have to retrain someone new, which takes time, but to me there is no other choice because of the time you save.

The place this is most evident is getting someone's bite perfect. The traditional way of measuring a bite to see if it is correct after a procedure is to have the patient bite down on an impressionable piece of paper. Of course this is not always 100% accurate and is also the main reason why these procedures take so long from start to finish.

I use a digital bite recorder, which takes an actual recording of someone's bite with 1600 sensors to tell me exactly what point of their bite is hitting first so that I can make any adjustments necessary. This saves a lot of time and discomfort for the patient.

All of these things come together to make the procedures I deliver the fastest in the business, the most accurate in the business, and the most aesthetic in the business. Because these technologies don't just allow me to move more quickly, they allow me to focus on the quality of the work.

It's very important that you never compromise for speed, but that doesn't mean you can't do things very quickly. You just have to be willing to pay for these materials and technologies that are so much more expensive and care enough to be up to date on what's out there.

When I do a repair on my hand drill the repair costs as much as most other dentists' entire drill costs. But I don't care. I know no one wants to sit there and listen to a drill for hours and hours. Why would you put someone through that when you can cut it down by so much?

Chapter 7

Pain Free Dentistry

Having established himself as a "Pain Free Dentist" over a decade ago, Dr. Maddahi goes over what discoveries have allowed him to push towards the eradication of dental phobia, and what it takes to make the procedures delivered in dentistry much less painful.

§

I've been a cosmetic dentist for over 27 years, and in that time I have noticed many shortcomings in my field.

The one I have come across most frequently is that dentistry is almost always associated with pain, and because of this people dread the dentist. In pop culture this can be easily observed with sayings like, "It was worse than a root canal."

It has always been my goal to observe any given situation in my life and see where I can improve it, nowhere more than in the level of service available to my patients. So in the beginning of my career I set out to first pinpoint what about dental work was so painful for people and second, how I could change it. Here's what I have found.

There are 3 things that cause distress and pain for the majority of the patients that sit in my chair:

1. The injection of anesthetics

2. The noise of the drill

3. The drilling itself

Numbing

The first thing to be addressed was the administering of anesthetics. In most anesthetics there is a chemical called epinephrine which causes a burning sensation, and this is the source of most of the pain one experiences when receiving an injection. So I started introducing a topical anesthetic to numb the gums before the local anesthetic and also trying an anesthetic that didn't have the epinephrine.

The upshot to epinephrine, however, is that it keeps the anesthetic in one spot for longer, so using the anesthetic that didn't have it meant that I would have to administer it more frequently. Or I would have to take three steps: topical anesthetic, followed by the anesthetic without epinephrine, followed by the regular anesthetic.

I also discovered that the slower the anesthetic was delivered the less painful it was, so I began using a delivery system where the anesthetic would slowly drip through for the patient.

All of these things made the numbing process much more thorough, but I wanted to streamline it, so I started using a machine called Air-Abrasion which used a combination of aluminum oxide powder and air to remove tooth structure. This machine caused no pain for the patient, so no anesthetic was needed, and it doesn't make noise like a hand drill, which also helps make the experience more tolerable, but it could only remove fairly shallow cavities, and the powder was very messy.

The system I moved to next is the one I still use today, which is one I have covered previously, and that is laser technology, which relieves the need for so many anesthetics and cancels out the noise of the drill as a factor in discomfort as well.

As the lasers that come out become stronger and more accurate, there's no telling what advancements we will be able to make with them, and I am a strong advocate of their use in all the medical fields.

Noise

The next thing, and probably the simplest to fix, is the noise of the drill. It is very difficult for people to sit for hours listening to a drill in their mouths. It causes many of my patients just as much discomfort as the pain one might experience from a shot.

Early on in my career I started setting up my patients with headphones or 3D glasses so that they could watch movies during procedures. This made the whole process much more relaxing for them and made it feel like their time in the chair was moving by more quickly, since they weren't just staring at me or the ceiling for hours.

Drills

Lastly is the drilling itself. There's not much that can be done about the discomfort of drilling, except to make sure you're using the absolutely fastest drill on the market, so as to move through the drilling as quickly as possible. I have always made sure that I do this by using the best electric hand drill and the best burrs that are available today.

All of these things combine to make dental procedures nearly painless, which is how one earns the title of a "Pain Free Dentist." It's one of my most coveted titles because it means that people won't dread coming into my office, which is certainly something to smile about.

Chapter 8

Dentistry From the Outside In: Case Studies

The following are accounts of several cases of patients who received Anti-Aging Dentistry procedures that were life changing. The patients whose stories are told here are thanked for their cooperation and enthusiasm for Dr. Maddahi and the work they had done.

§

The first patient I want to talk about is Nancy, who was my most recent large-scale case. The thing about Nancy is that she is a very beautiful woman, and looking at her one wouldn't think that she needed any work done, but she had a growing concern about the lower part of her face. It seemed to be changing very rapidly.

She was beginning to consider different kinds of procedures to fix what was happening. I'm glad she came to see me first because the kinds of procedures she was considering wouldn't have solved the problems that were arising, and she would have ended up doing a lot of unnecessary and invasive things.

When I sit down in front of a patient for the first time, I'm looking at their entire face. I'm not looking at their teeth. All I'm interested in at the initial meeting are their facial features and facial structures, and I start to look at the flaws that I see in them. From that point I try to figure out if any of what I'm seeing could be caused by something going on inside of their mouth.

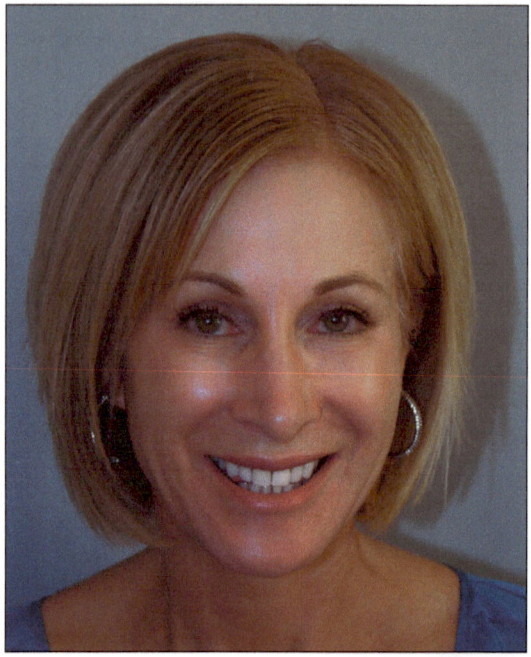

Patient Nancy Before

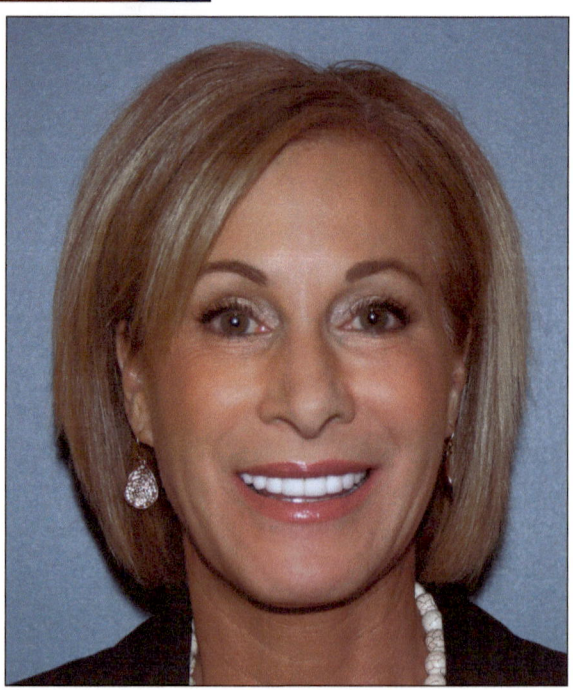

Patient Nancy After

So with Nancy I could see right away that the right side of her face went in farther than the left side. I saw a line on the side of her lip (which is commonly known as a laugh line) that was deeper on the left side than the right side. I saw two white horizontal lines right by the corners of her lips that were pretty deep. And I also saw that the upper lip was thinner than the lower lip.

The lower 1/3 of her face did not match the upper 2/3, and that was how I knew what was occurring most probably stemmed from what was going on inside her mouth.

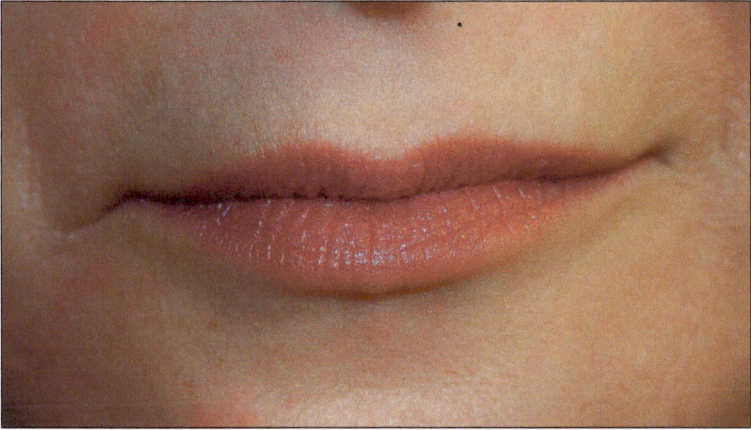

Upper Lip Before

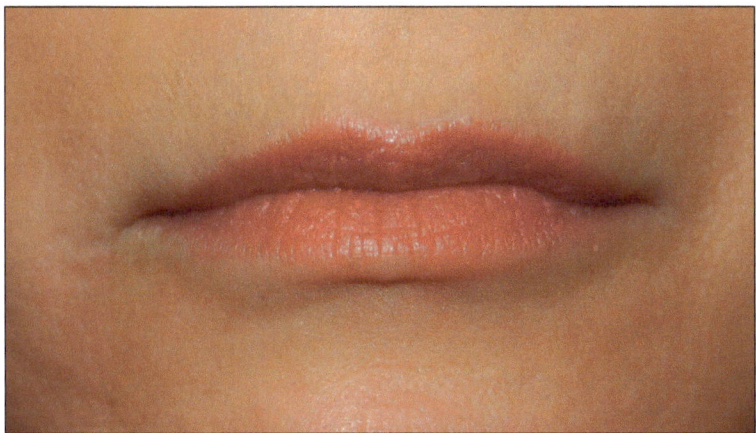

Upper Lip After

She then started to tell me that she had noticed a big change in her jaw line. She felt it had been changing a lot over the span of a year, and there was something about her face that was just not right now. She didn't know what had happened to create that effect.

I took a look at her jaw line and noticed that the skin there was hanging over a bit, and her chin was coming forward more than it should.

I recorded all of this in my mind, so when I started to do the exam I wasn't just looking at her teeth and her arch, I was looking specifically for the explanations for these issues.

The first thing I did was to tell her to smile. I immediately got two answers. I could see that her front teeth were tilted inwards. What does that tell you? That tells you right away why the upper lip was thinner than the lower lip and why the nose was being pulled down as the lip disappeared. There was a lack of support.

Next I asked her to smile bigger, and when she did I could see that the right side of her jaw was going in farther than the left side. This explained why the right side of her face was more sunken in than the left side. There was something structurally wrong that was creating this symmetrical problem.

Overall the jaw was narrow, and when I looked inside her mouth I could see her entire upper arch was narrow. Many people that have had orthodontic treatments in the past where teeth have been extracted to help with crowding have this issue. When the Orthodontist closes those gaps that are created by the extracted teeth, the arch becomes very narrow.

This used to be a very common way of trying to handle overcrowded teeth, and it causes quite a few very distinct wrinkles and lines to appear in someone's face over time.

Restoring Youth, One Smile at a Time

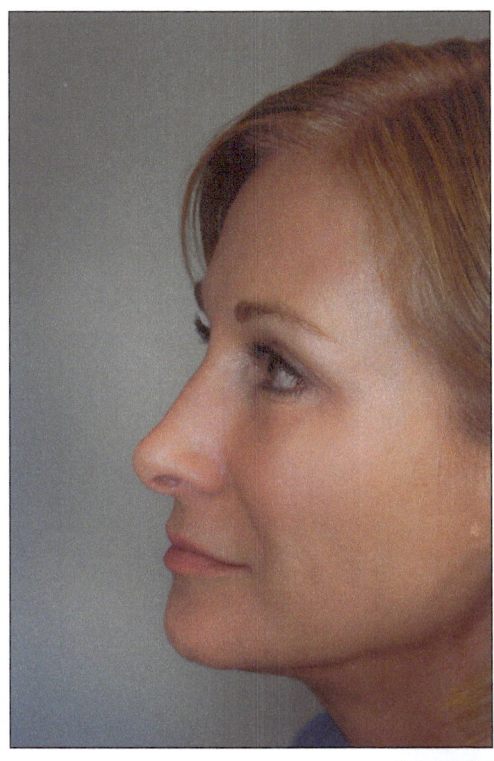

Nancy's Chin Before

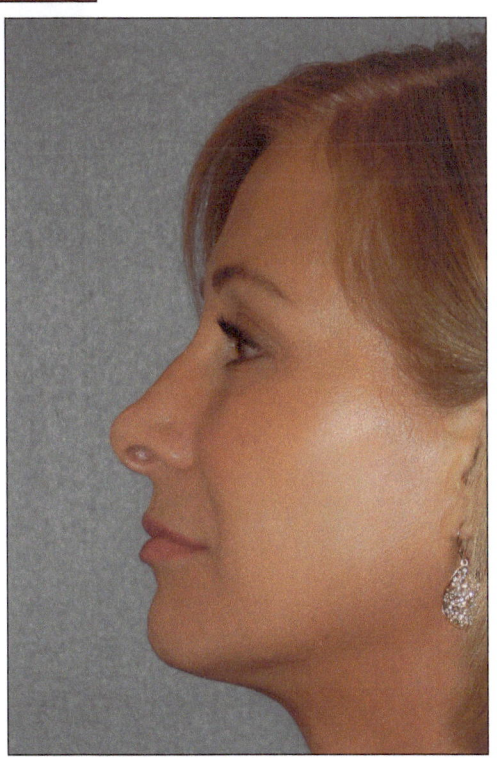

Nancy's Chin After

Orthodontists that are knowledgeable about aesthetics, arch design, and bite don't do this anymore. It was a way to avoid having to widen the arch. In reality there are very few instances where taking teeth out because of overcrowding is a good solution.

Next were the lines in the corner of her lips, which were caused by her bite being too far closed. This is also what was making her chin come out too far, causing it to not be at a proper angle with the nose and lips.

Ideally the nose should come out farther than the lips, and the lips should come out farther than the chin, not the other way around.

When you open your mouth you can feel your chin go backward, and as you close your mouth you can feel it come forward. You only see this problem where someone's chin is jutting out past the correct point when the teeth have been worn down, allowing the bite to close more, which pushes the chin out.

At this point I knew more work needed to be done than what we initially talked about. At first we had just talked about doing some veneers on her bottom teeth because they were crooked and maybe a couple of the top teeth to give her more support for her lip, but after seeing everything else that was going on, and how much of her face it was affecting, more just had to be done.

I was going to have to open up the bite by lengthening the teeth, as well as build them out to give her back the width she needed in her arch. That was the only way I was going to be able to correct what was happening and handle everything that had changed in her face.

I was looking for the clues on the outside that would tell me what needed to be done inside. This is a new way of approaching dentistry. In the past dentistry was simply based on what was going on inside the mouth, but that's not even half of the puzzle.

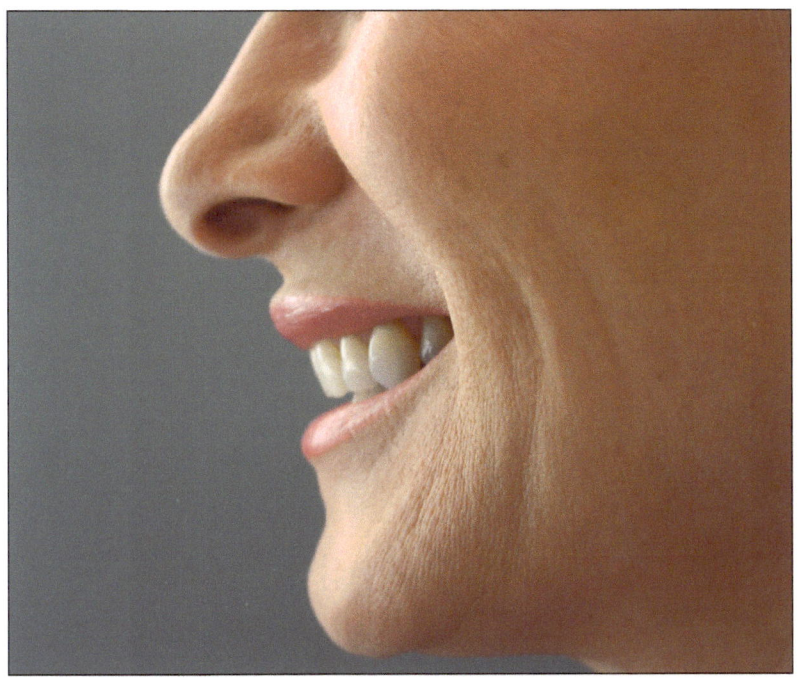
Teeth Tilted in from the Side Before

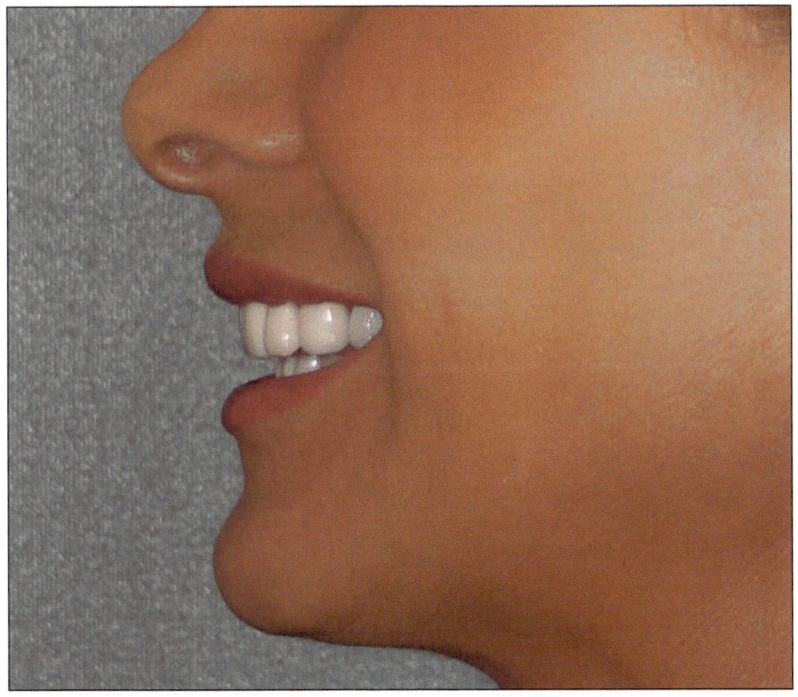
Teeth Tilted in from the Side After

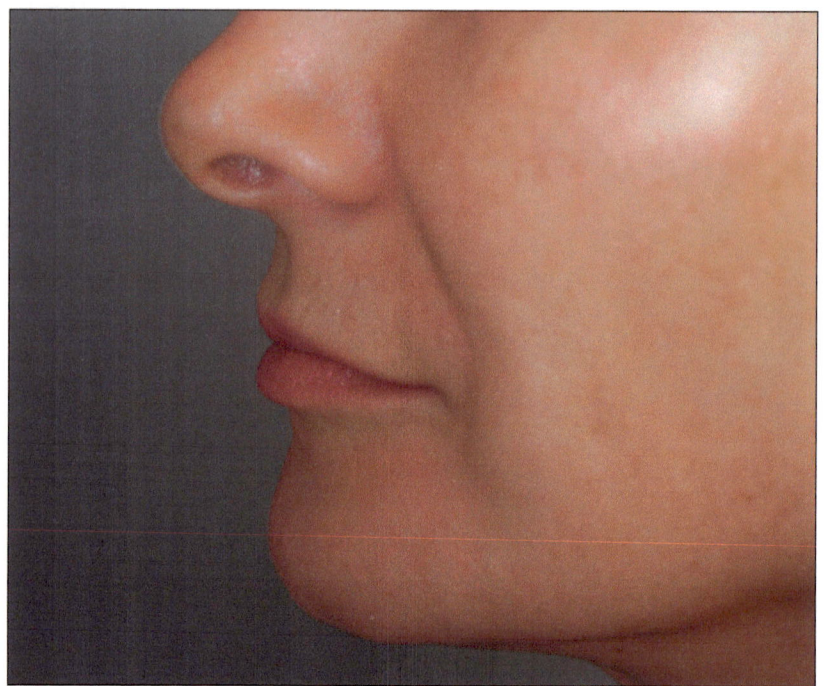

Incorrect Chin Angle

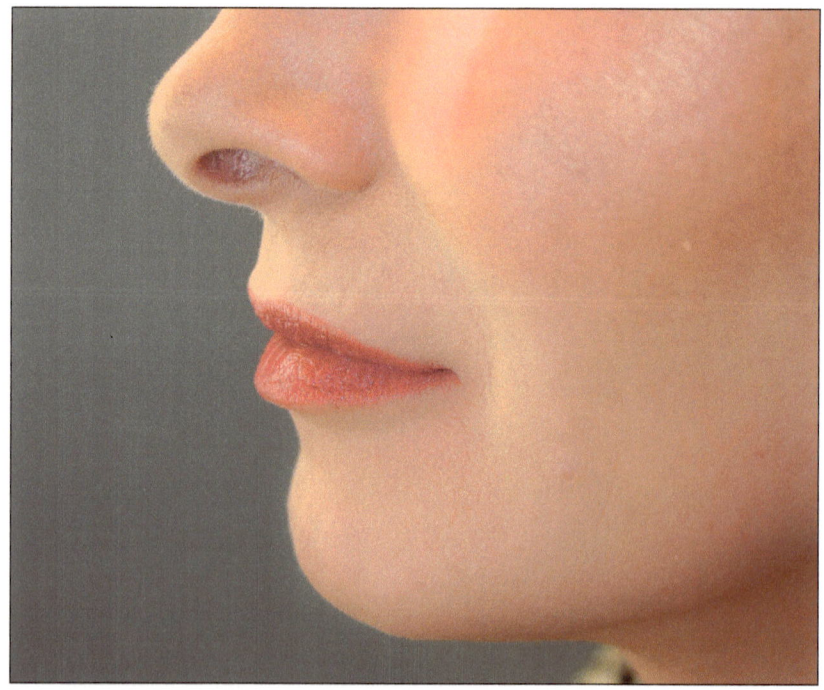

Chin Angle Corrected

This is why when I do cases like these my patient's end up looking 10 to 20 years younger. It will appear as if they had a facelift, because really that is what I'm doing. I'm lifting the face by building out the structure, and the effects will last so much longer because the support is from inside.

On a side note, Nancy was also complaining to me about these bumps that had appeared on the side of her lips. I asked her if she had ever gotten any kind of injections, and after thinking about it, she said yes.

There was a period of time not too long ago that more permanent injections were very popular. These particular kinds of injections get integrated into the tissues of a lot of people's faces, and they stayed there and hardened, which created these kinds of bumps.

I do not recommend those kinds of long-lasting or "permanent" injections. If you're going to get injections it's better that you get something that your body can actually get rid of.

The patients of mine that have suffered the most with lip movement, lost elasticity in the lips, or the appearance of these kinds of bumps all have long-lasting injections in common.

I could do a lot for Nancy, and in truth she probably wouldn't have needed much in the way of injections after I had done what needed to be done for her lips, but I can't reverse those kinds of bumps. So I do warn people against these kinds of "permanent" injectables. You think you're all set and that seems great, but what does "all set" mean?

Chapter 9

Tetracycline Stains

The next kind of case is one that has a particular kind of staining that I have worked for many years to be able to correct, and that is Tetracycline stains.

These are intrinsic stains that occur when someone has taken Tetracycline (a very effective antibiotic prescribed for fevers) as a child before the teeth are fully developed. The staining is usually a dark grayish-brown and because it is under the enamel of the tooth, in most cases it is impossible to treat without the use of veneers or crowns.

The majority of these patients have either been turned away by other dentists who did not want to remove unnecessary tooth structure or have had veneers and crowns put on, but the stains have begun to show through the porcelain.

The people who have Tetracycline stains have typically felt held back by the appearance of their smile their entire adult lives. That is worth handling.

For example, recently a young medical student came in to see me who had darker stains than is normal because he also had a condition called Amelogenesis imperfecta where the teeth grow in with no enamel, so there was nothing to mask the stains.

Anti-Aging Dentistry

Because there was missing enamel his teeth were also thinner than normal, giving him very little support for his upper lip. He was too young to be seeing much of an adverse effect in his face from this, but I knew if I widened the arch by building his teeth out he wouldn't see the aging effects of it in the future.

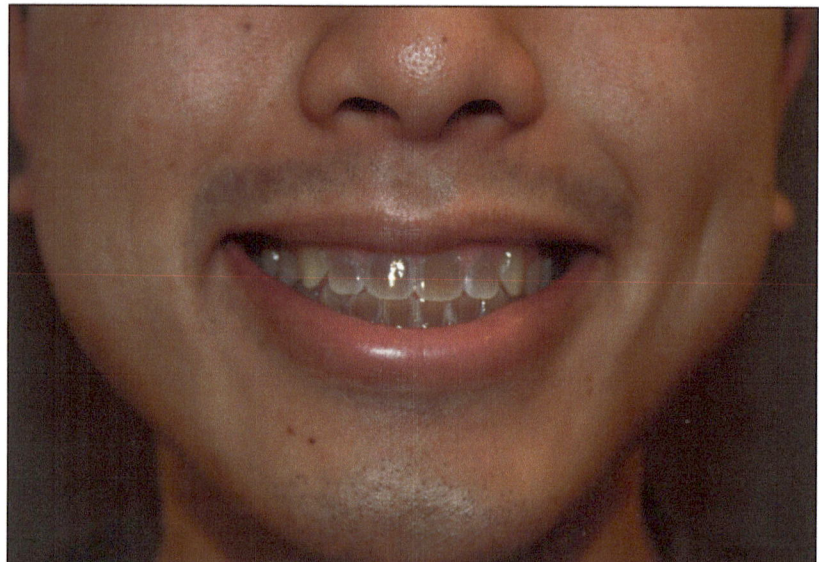

Patient Julien Before

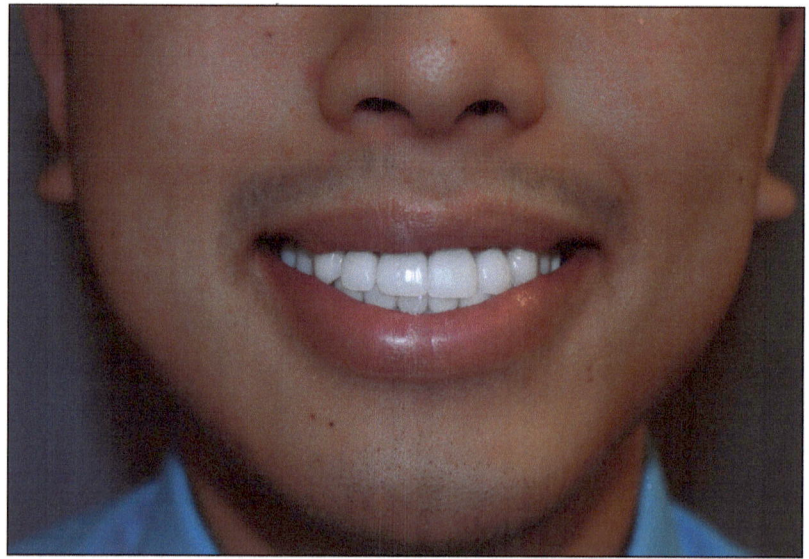

Patient Julien After

There was another complicating factor in this case. He had just graduated from a very prestigious medical school and was about to start his career the next week, so he only had 5 days to do this.

That's not at all unheard of for me, but it was something to consider, and he, being in medicine himself, had very high expectations. He had done a lot of research about what he wanted done.

This is great in one way, but it can sometimes be a hindrance because what "can be done" and what I can do are usually two different things. It took me quite a while to convince him of what I thought he needed, even though he believed I was the absolute best guy to do the job.

He had also been told by many of the other specialists he had talked to through the years that he would have to get a mouth full of crowns. This is a very common misconception with Tetracycline stains, which is also one of the reasons many dentists try to persuade people away from doing this kind of work, suggesting they try and live with the stains if they can.

In dentistry it is absolute blasphemy to remove tooth structure unnecessarily. It is looked down upon. But you do not need to do a full mouth of crowns in order to fix this problem. It took me many years of perfecting the way I do these procedures, but after so many of them I have been able to pin point the exact amount of tooth structure that needs to be taken away, and thus am able to get the job done with veneers instead of crowns (which requires less tooth structure removal).

In the end we were able to do something that he didn't think was possible. The teeth were longer than he originally had thought they should be, they were built out farther than he had anticipated, and they were whiter than he had thought they should be. All of that being said, when it was all done he told me he couldn't believe what he saw when he looked in the mirror. It had given him the smile he had always dreamed of having, but really didn't think could ever be. He was so happy because he really felt he was going to be able to go into his new profession with a smile that people would trust.

Smiles are very important for trust. In fact, there have been many studies that show that people who have crooked or stained teeth appear to be less trustworthy. And, of course, when you're going into the medical field, the last thing you want to have is distrust. It's so important that people feel safe with you.

The other Tetracycline case I'm going to talk about was interesting because she also had a ton of other issues in her mouth.

Since she was an older woman and had been living with the stains for so long, she had given up trying to take care of them after years of feeling that nothing she did made a difference.

This happens with many of the severe cases that come in to see me. There's something wrong with their teeth, and no matter how well they take care of them nothing changes that, so they give up completely, and then the teeth really start to fall apart.

This was the case with my patient Kim. She came in with her husband to see me right before the holidays. She hadn't had any hope that anything could be done about her teeth for many years, but she was starting to have pain in her back teeth now and she needed to revisit the entire subject.

This is when she found my website, and she started looking at some before and after photos I have there. She began to have hope again that maybe something could be done.

Restoring Youth, One Smile at a Time

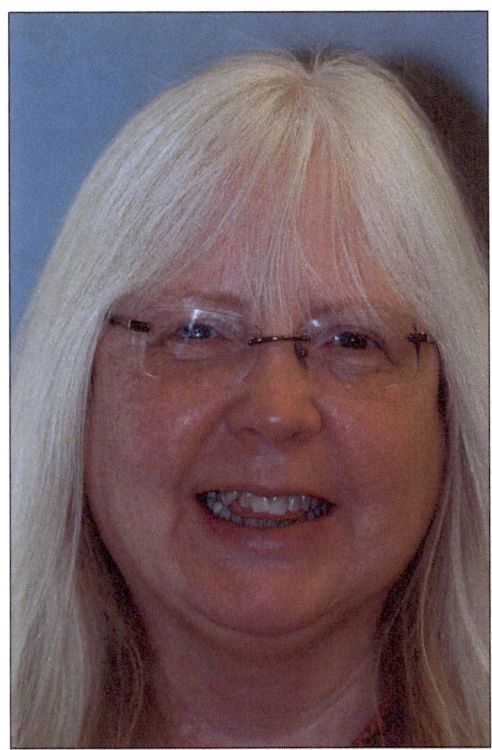

Patient Kim Before

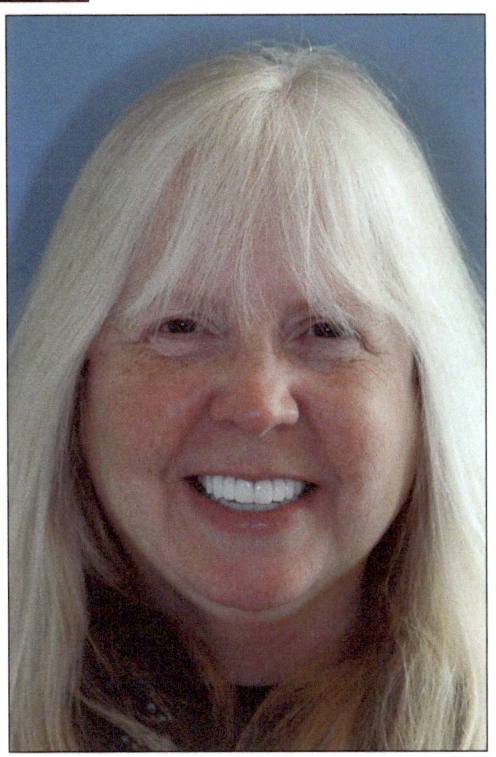

Patient Kim After

Chapter 9: Tetracycline Stains

She came in to see me, and even though the pain in her back teeth was what had spurred the initial search, she told me she really didn't care about that.

After seeing the photos on my website she just wanted to know if anything could be done about her front teeth.

Of course there was, but I explained to her that we had to take care of her back teeth first because there was quite a bit of decay, and she would need to have some root canals done before I could do anything else.

She had a level of fear of the dentist that was paralyzing. It isn't terribly common that I come across a patient who is so afraid that they almost can't get any of the work done. But this was the case with Kim.

Once she came back from her root canals and we started to talk about what we were going to do, it was very clear that I was going to need to put her under for both the temporaries and for the final cementation.

The good thing about this was I knew it was going to really change her life. She was going to go to sleep, and when she woke up her teeth would be fixed.

When she woke up from the cementation, her teeth were so perfect and beautiful she started sobbing immediately. She really couldn't believe that she had waited for so many years to have this done.

She told me that she had completely isolated herself over recent years. She had stopped smiling, and she avoided talking much because of her teeth.

Now she felt like she could laugh again without having to be self-conscious about what people were going to think about her smile. She went to sleep, woke up, and just like that, she had her life back.

Chapter 10
Quality of Life

There's another kind of patient that I want to address. This is a purely cosmetic case. This is someone who does not have a dental need to get work done.

I have one case that I just started to work on that's the perfect example of this.

A woman named Kathy saw the CBS special on Nancy and had been noticing a drastic change in her own face over a 6-month period. The lines in her face had been getting much deeper and the lower 1/3 seemed to be collapsing.

She had been very bothered by this, but none of the professionals she had gone to see could give her a solution to it because there was no obvious dental need for a procedure, but she was miserable. She felt that something was wrong with her face, and it seemed to be getting worse. Rapidly.

The entire problem with Kathy has nothing to do with dentistry, but it has everything to do with dentistry, and when she saw that program on CBS and saw that something could be done she was blown away. She contacted my office immediately, because finally what she was saying was understood. Someone got what was bothering her so much, that she hadn't been able to find a solution for.

This is what sets Anti-Aging Dentistry apart. It's long term, and it has a broad focus. Cosmetic Dentistry is limited to the teeth, where Anti-Aging Dentistry is taking on the entire lower part of the face.

The quality of someone's life is what I'm paying attention to in these cases. Kathy wasn't in any physical pain, but she had lost confidence in her smile and had a growing concern about the changes she was seeing. And that is another kind of pain that I often take just as seriously as physical pain because it's stopping someone from living his or her life fully.

I have patients who come in to see me and say they don't leave the house, or they try not to smile. It is very painful for them.

One perfect example of this kind of case is a man who came in to see me a few years ago named Ted who was 88 years old. He had a denture that he had been living with for quite a few years, and it had created some bone loss for him, which made the denture a little loose. He wanted to have implants put in.

I asked him why he would want to do something like that at that stage in his life. It's quite a lot of work to put in that many implants and everything, and do you know what he said to me?

'I just want to be able to eat a hot dog again.'

That's when I understood that this man's quality of life had been compromised. He could no longer eat a hot dog or hamburger and enjoy it, and it was really important to him. I said 'Okay! Let's do it then.' And his mouth fell open.

He said, 'You know, everyone else that I have told has laughed at me.'

But I got it. These are the things in our lives that make life worth

Restoring Youth, One Smile at a Time

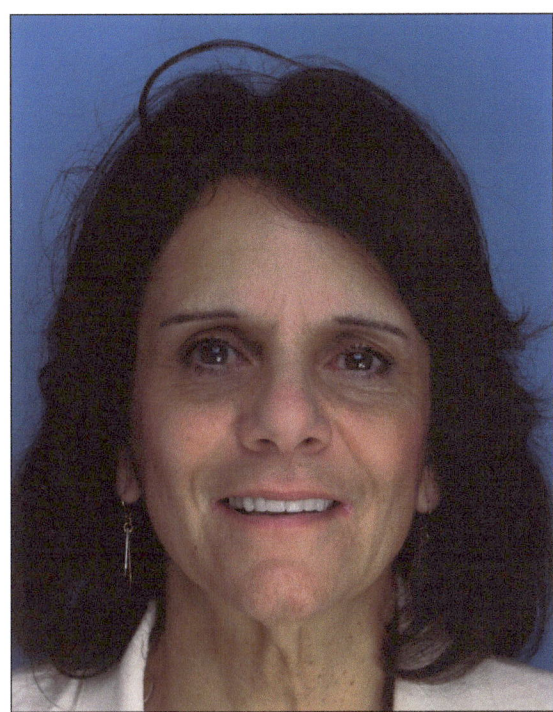

Patient Kathy Before

Patient Kathy After

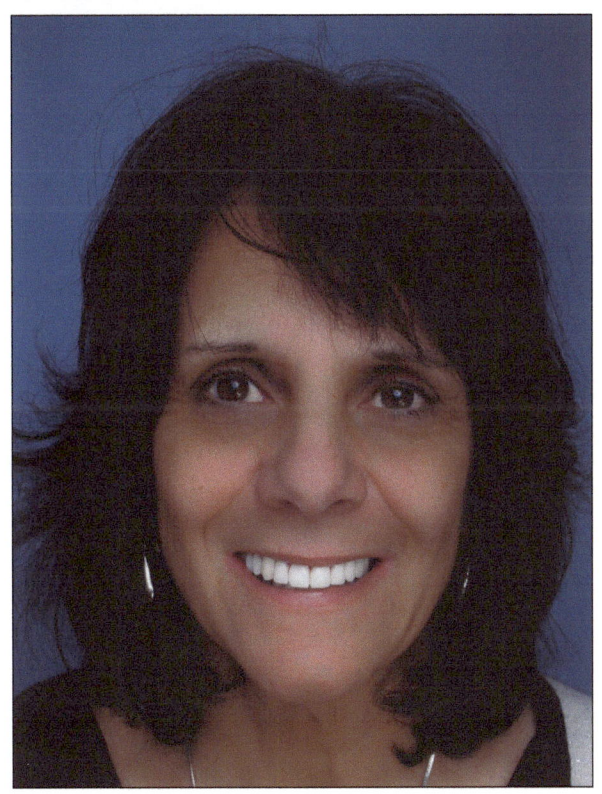

living, and I don't think anyone at any age should be robbed of that. So, we went ahead and started doing the work and getting the implants put in, and when everything was done he had a full set of teeth.

That night when I was at home around 7:30 or 8 I got a call on my home phone. There he was on the other end, 'Hey doc! It's me, Ted! I just wanted to tell you where I am. I'm at a hot dog stand with my girlfriend and I'm eating a hot dog, and I'm so happy. This is the best day of my life. You gave me my dream.'

I was so pleased, because I knew it was his quality of life that was important.

There's another case like this I had several years ago. A woman came in to see me who was 91. She had gotten implants when that was a completely new technology in the late 50s. The technology was not very good then and most of those implants came out or needed to be removed at some point over the years, but hers hadn't.

This woman was exceptional. I remember the way she looked very well. She really took care of herself. She got her nails done 2 or 3 times a week, she had her hair done every single day, and her clothes were perfectly pressed. She really cared about those kinds of things.

When she came in to see me and told me she needed to have these implants replaced, I asked her if she wouldn't prefer to have a denture made, but that was out of the question for her. She shook her head and said firmly 'no'. She didn't want to have anything removable in her mouth. She didn't care if she was only alive for another 6 months, she told me, she wanted to live the way she wanted to live, and that was that.

I didn't see the point in fighting her on it, so we did it. It was a very long process because there was a lot of infection from the old implants

Restoring Youth, One Smile at a Time

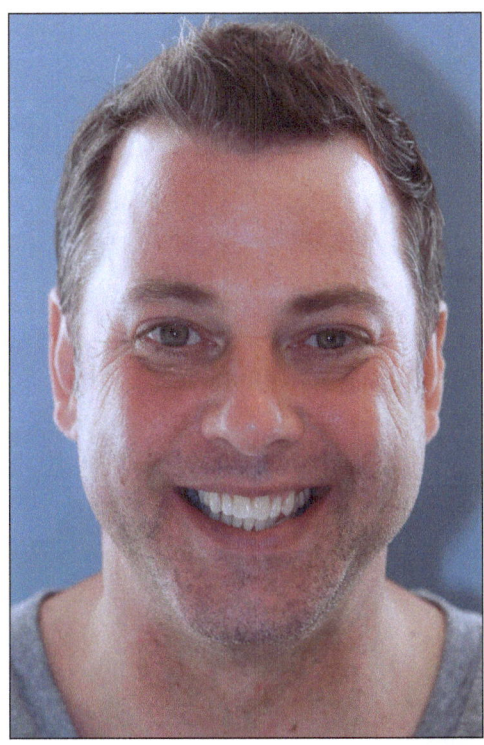

Patient Michael Before

Patient Michael After

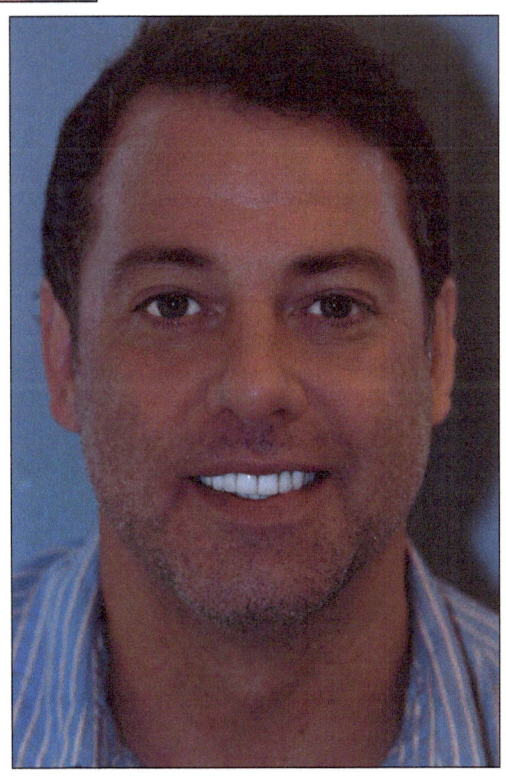

Chapter 10: Quality of Life

that had to be handled and we had to grow new bone because there was quite a bit missing. In the end she had exactly what she wanted and they looked really great.

The one other case that comes to mind that is kind of related to this was a man named Michael. He came in to my office with his girlfriend one day to talk about getting a full mouth reconstruction. He explained to me that he had started to notice that his teeth were not that great at a fairly young age, and no matter how many times he whitened them he couldn't get them to look how he wanted them to, so he had sort of given up on them.

He explained to me that he didn't really know what it was about his smile that bothered him, but he had never liked it and he hated looking at pictures of himself.

This was a patient who really didn't have anything medically wrong with him, but he was so self-conscious about his smile that it was affecting his social life and even his confidence level at work. As a young man he had been a great athlete so feeling this way was not something that he was used to, and it was really bothering him.

I have spent a lot of time looking at different smiles and studying the ones that are renowned for being beautiful. I have spent hours looking at Julia Roberts' smile or Halle Berry's smile to find out what it is about them that people love so much, and one of the things that I have found is that the width of the smile line has a lot to do with it.

As we have previously covered, if someone has a narrow arch they are going to have dark holes in the sides of their cheeks. This doesn't look nearly as good as someone who does not have them. I told Michael that this was the main reason he did not like his smile, coupled with the shape of his teeth and the color. I had him smile and pointed these dark spots out and he immediately got what I was talking about.

Restoring Youth, One Smile at a Time

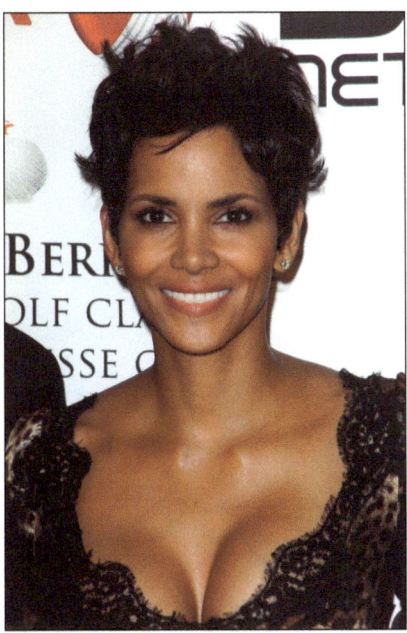

Actress Halle Berry

His reaction to the final product of the work we did stuck with me for a long time.

When we were done with Michael's teeth, and he saw his new smile for the first time he just started sobbing. He told me he never thought he could have this. He said he actually looked *more* like himself.

This transformation gave him the confidence he had experienced as a young athlete. He felt newly energized. It made a huge difference with the way he felt about his own appearance, how he presented himself in social settings, and how he interacted in business.

These are the kinds of cases that make me so glad I do what I do. I can make that big of a difference in someone's life by giving him or her a real change that they wouldn't be able to get anywhere else.

Chapter 11

Self Evaluation

Dr. Maddahi walks you through how to spot the abnormalities in the mouth and jaw that can be corrected by Anti-Aging Dentistry.

§

So now that I've explained some of my cases and what can be done in terms of this kind of work, I want to explain how one can look in the mirror or at pictures and spot if any of these types of problems are occurring in their own face.

Lips

Let's start with the lips. Look at them with your mouth closed and relaxed to see if the upper and lower lips are really symmetrical. Is the same amount showing?

If your upper lip is in fact thinner than your lower lip, then you can look at a profile photo of yourself while you're smiling to see if your teeth are straight up and down or tilting in.

Next you want to check if you have lines in the corners of your lips. If you do have lines, your jaw is too far closed, which is creating a squished look in the lower part of your face.

Anti-Aging Dentistry

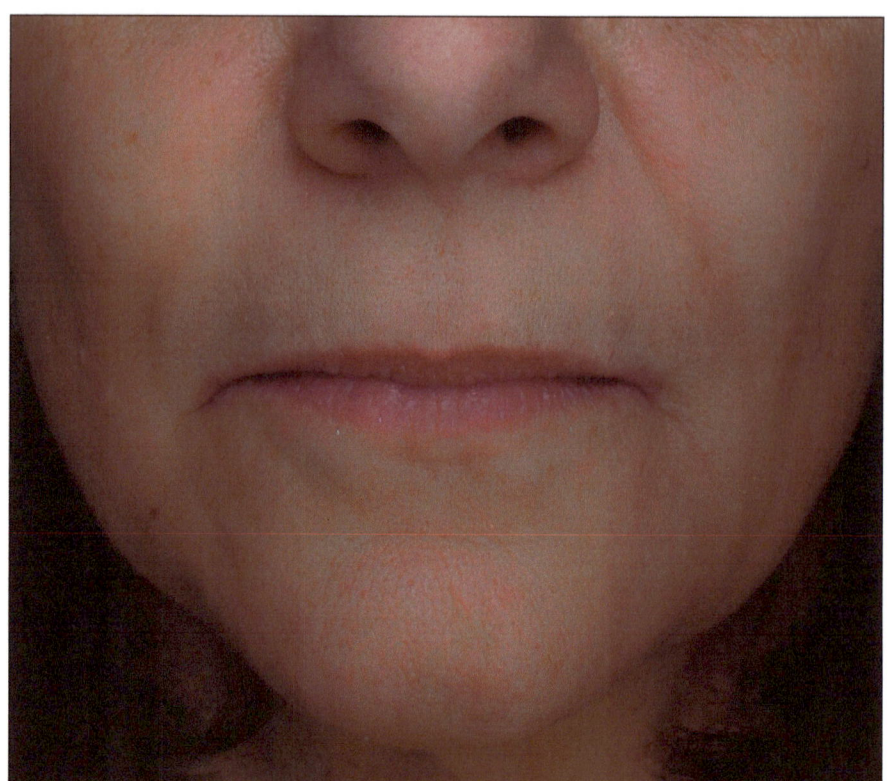

Uneven Lip

Now, if there are these kinds of lines and the bite is not corrected by lengthening the teeth, they will continue to get deeper over time as more wearing occurs.

After that what you want to look at is if you have vertical wrinkles on the lips. This can stem from a lack of support causing the lips to thin out and lines to appear or from habits like smoking.

The next thing to look for requires a profile photo of yourself from the past and a current profile photo to see if your nose is coming down farther than it used to. If that is happening it is also because of the loss of support in your upper lip. When the lip thins out and starts to disappear it will pull the nose down as well.

Restoring Youth, One Smile at a Time

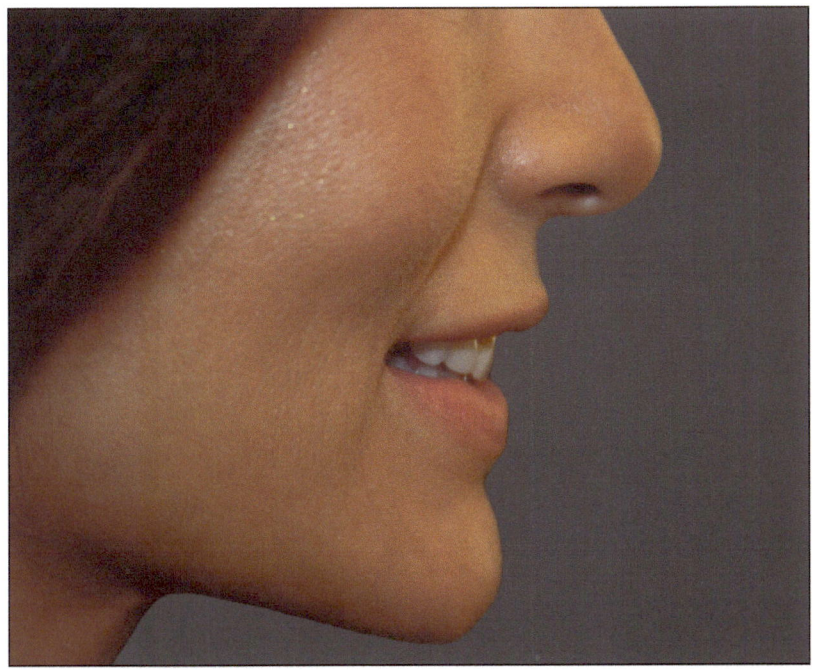

Tilted in Teeth Before

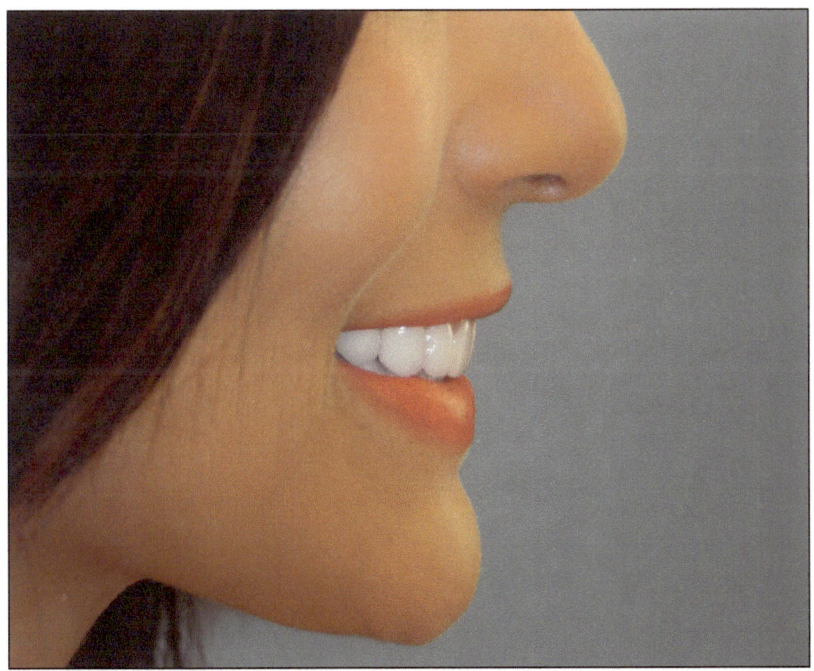

Tilted in Teeth After

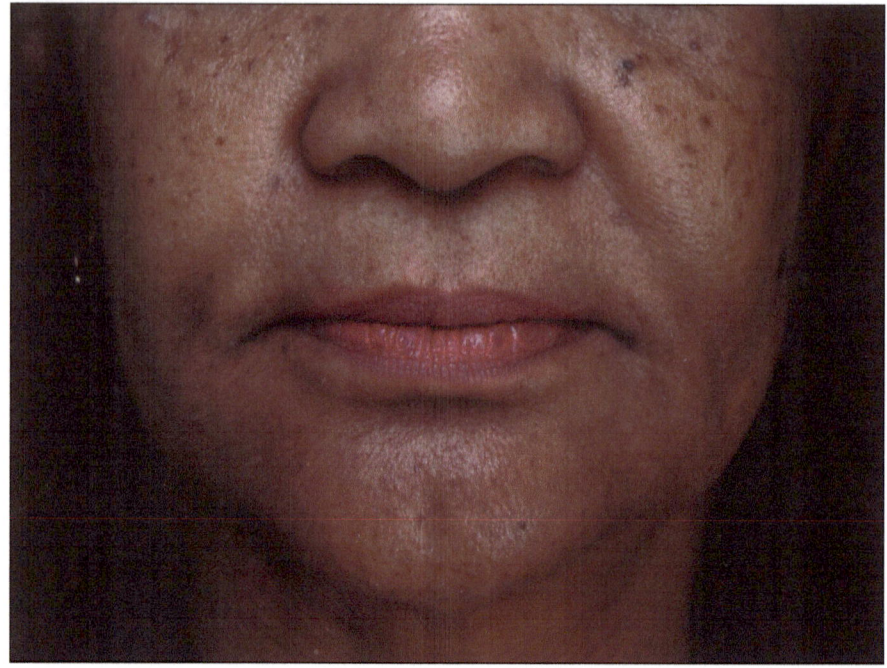
Squished Lower 1/3 of the Face Before

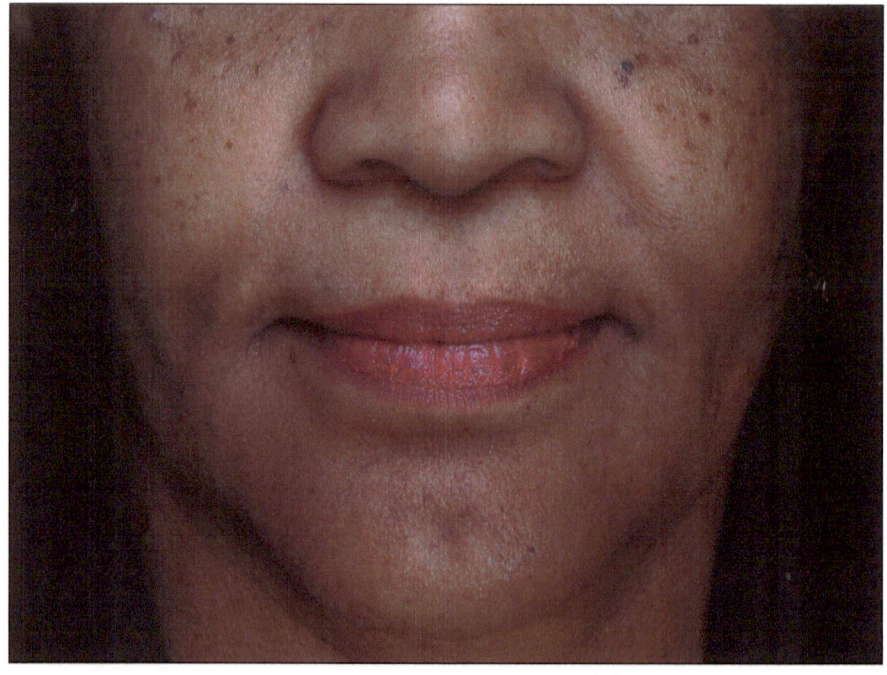
Squished Lower 1/3 of the Face After

Restoring Youth, One Smile at a Time

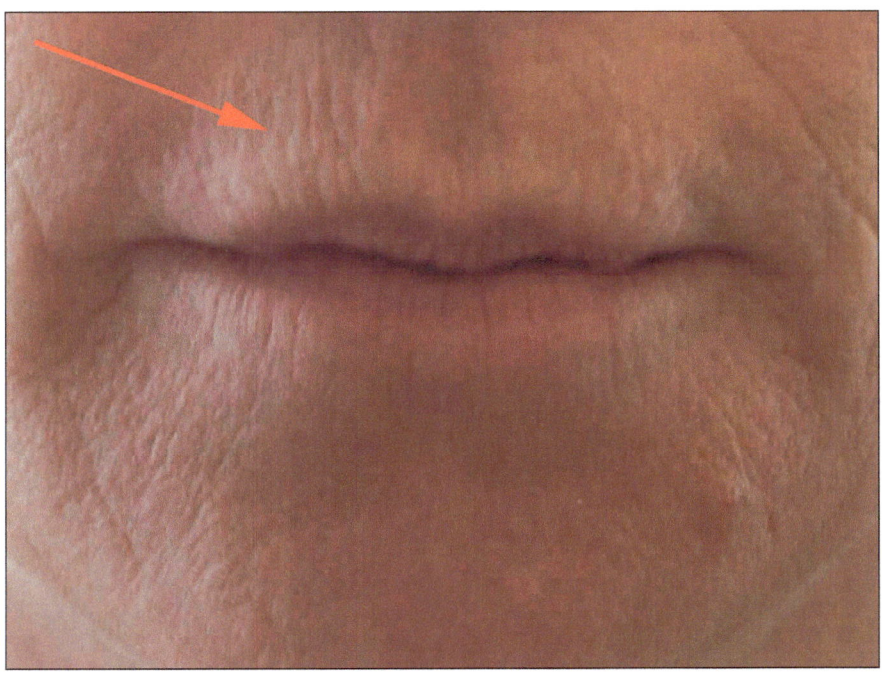

Lines Around the Lips Before

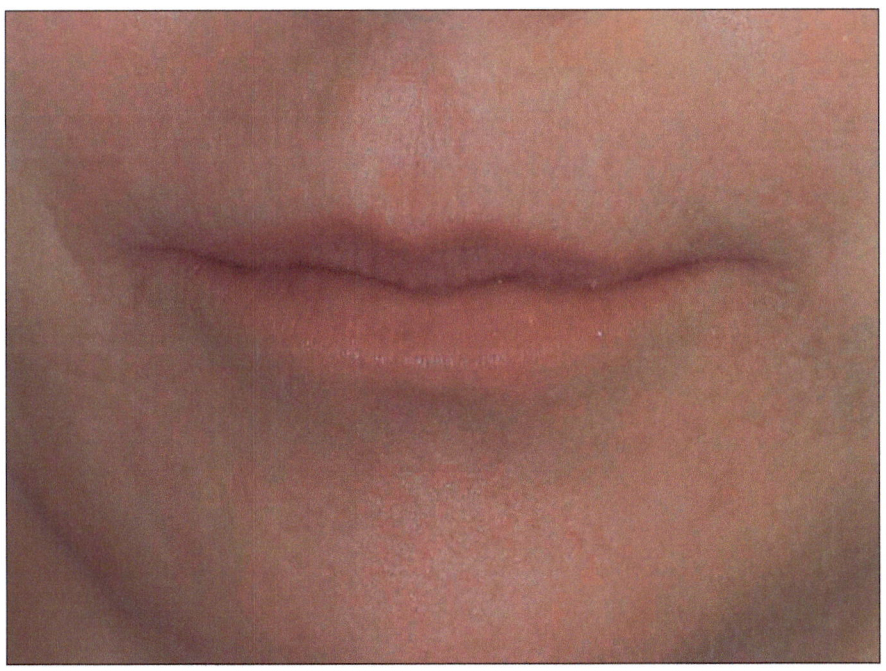

Lines Around the Lips After

Anti-Aging Dentistry

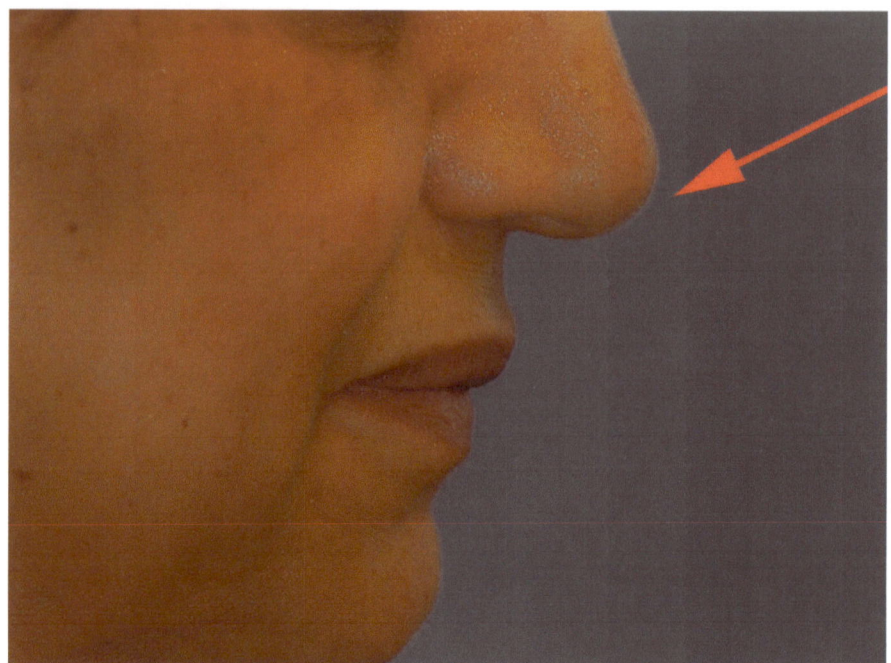

Nose Pulled Down

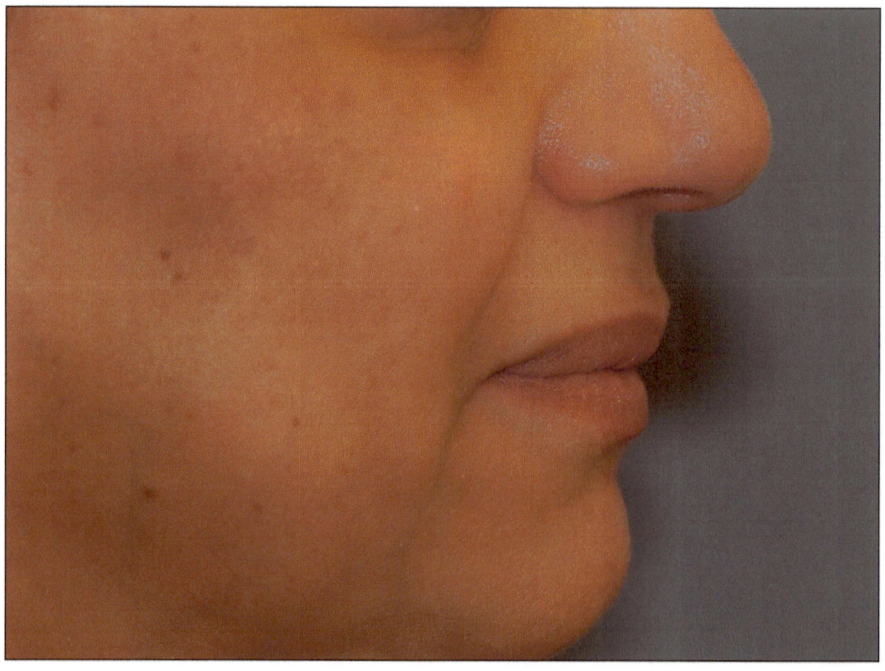

Nose in Correct Position

Teeth

Now let's take a look at the teeth. First you can check to see if your front teeth have any wear marks. This would tell you if your teeth have gotten shorter over time.

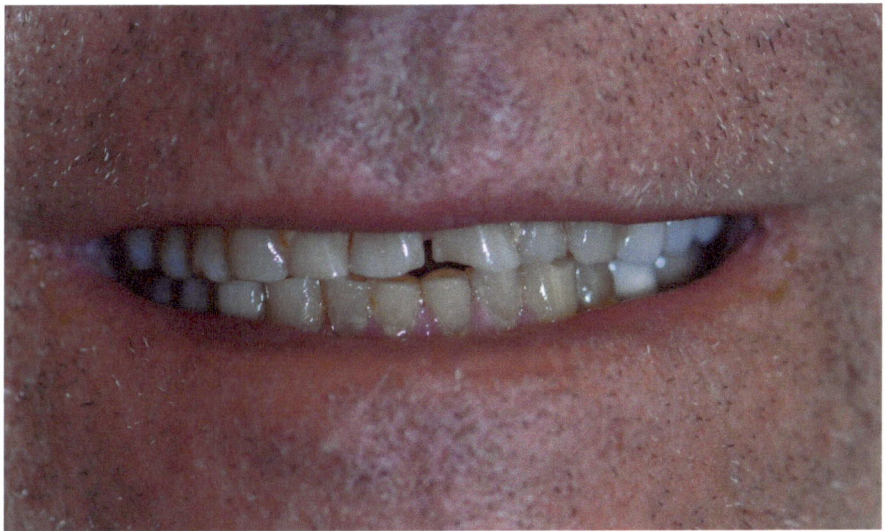

Front Teeth with Wear Marks from Grinding Before

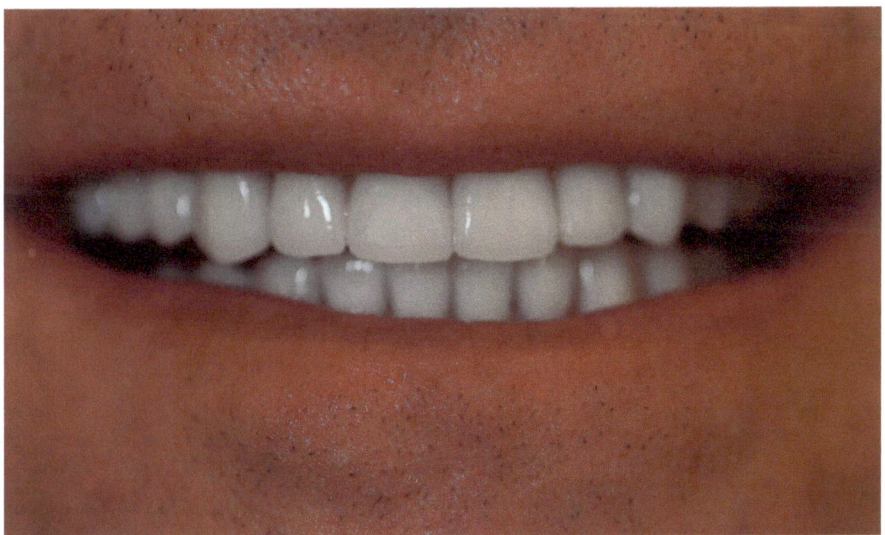

Front Teeth with Wear Marks from Grinding After

The other way to tell if your teeth have gotten shorter is to get an older photo of you where you are smiling and compare that smile to your smile today to see if your teeth have changed.

If they appear shorter or more crowded, these are signs that over a long period of time clenching and grinding or possibly eating a diet of hard foods has affected the shape of your entire mouth.

If it is clenching and grinding and it's happening at night (which is most likely), it will continue to get worse without the use of a night guard.

The next thing I would recommend doing is taking a few photos from the past where you're smiling and try to see if it looks as though your teeth are becoming more crooked over time.

If the teeth were straight 10 or 20 years ago and now they're not, that tells you that one of two things has happened. Either you had orthodontic work and maybe you didn't wear your retainer, or you clench and grind and all of the pressure that you're putting on your teeth is moving them slowly over time, and it will continue to get worse. Your teeth will bunch up more and more over time if you don't do something to change this pattern.

I have stressed this point a lot, but that is because this problem is the one that causes the most damage to not just your teeth, but also everything else that is connected to the lower 1/3 of your face.

You're putting your teeth in constant transition; they're moving, and this is changing the shape of the arch, the shape of the jaw, and the muscles surrounding it. The aging effects of this can creep up on you. When it starts to really show up in the face where you can see noticeable differences, everything else falls apart pretty quickly after that.

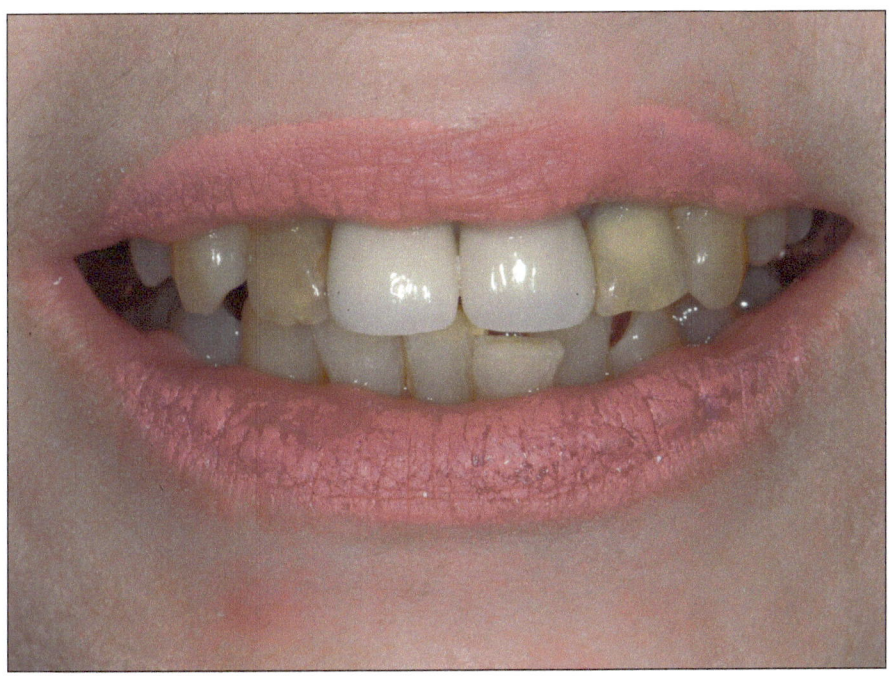

Teeth that Have Shifted Over Time Before

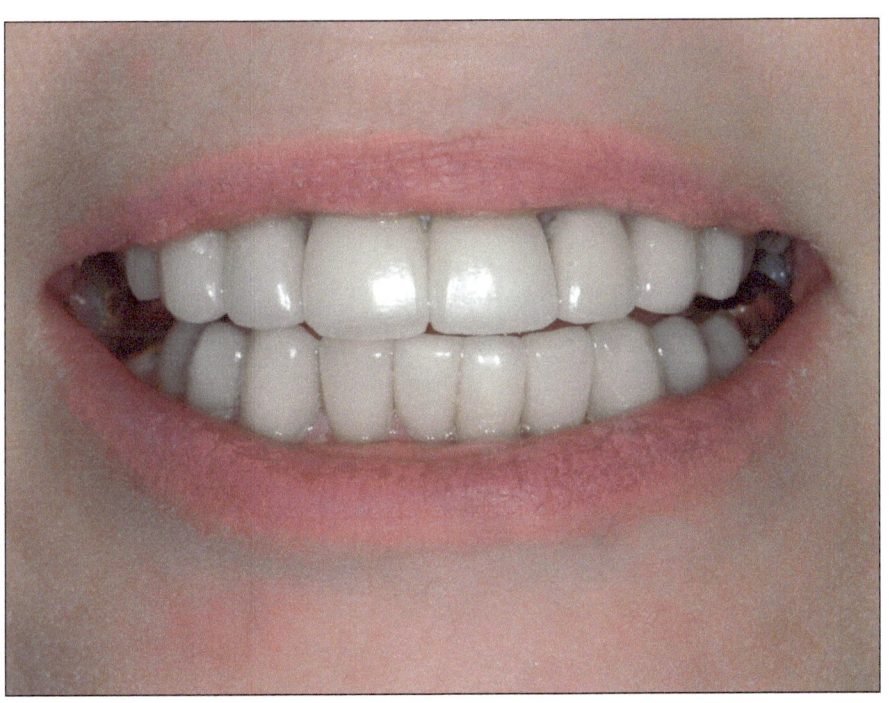

Teeth that Have Shifted Over Time After

So one day you may start to notice there's some unevenness going on in your lips and then in just a year or so your face is much more hollowed, you've lost support in your cheeks, and you feel as if you have aged 10 years.

This is why I so strongly urge my patients to pay attention to what they are doing with their jaw muscles throughout the day. Pay attention to how you feel when you wake up in the morning. Do you feel well rested, or do you always have a feeling of exhaustion following you around? If you do in fact clench and grind while you sleep, you are never actually entering an REM state, which can cause someone to feel like they never get enough rest.

Do you wake up with headaches or get them late in the afternoon? You may attribute this to stress, which is completely accurate, but where is that stress going? If you're holding it in your jaw by clenching or grinding your teeth together, you are wearing those teeth down and doing a lot of damage.

Arch

Next look in a mirror head on and smile. Do you see any black holes from the side of your teeth to your cheeks (like in Michael's case)? If you do it's because your arch is too narrow, and as you get older those black holes are going to get bigger because you're going to lose the fat inside your cheeks.

You can also compare your smile today to a past photo to see if those black spaces that you do have are getting any larger. If you didn't really have them before, but you do now, I can guarantee you that trend is going to continue.

Next, close your lips and see if one side of your face is going in farther than the other side of your face *or* if you feel that your lips are full on one side and then on the other side they're collapsing. This could be as a result of the arch not being wide enough as well.

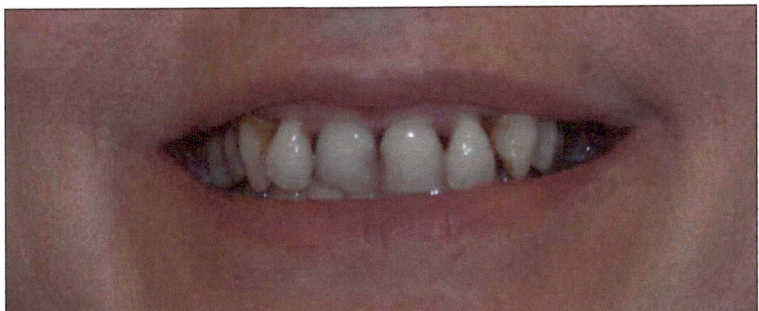

Smile with Black Holes Before

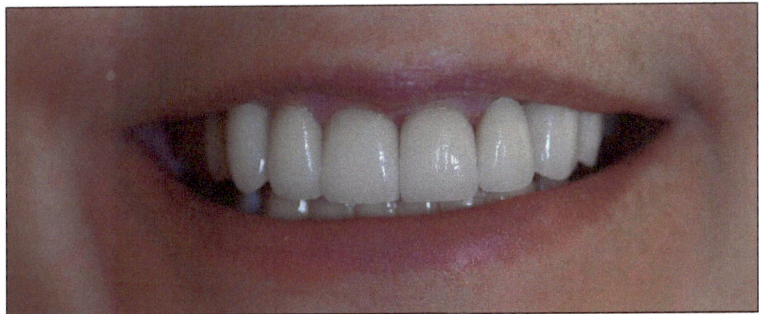

Smile with Black Holes After

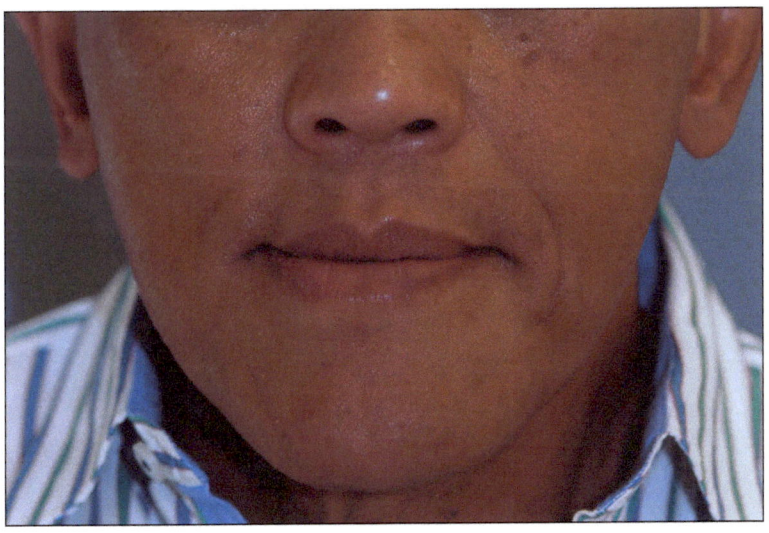

Uneven Face

The Root

It is important to be able to spot what is physically showing up on your face, but it is equally as important to be able to spot the habits and routines that cause these things. If you do not treat something from the root of the problem, you will not be able to handle it properly or for very long.

That's why I don't always look at someone's teeth when I'm trying to figure out what I can do for them. I don't always need to. I can see exactly what is going on based on these elements around the lips and cheeks.

To determine if you are a clencher and grinder or not, you can look at yourself in the mirror with your lips closed and pay attention to the jaw line and the muscle of the jaw from the ear all the way to the middle of the jaw line. Looking at those muscles, you may be able to see if they are sticking out slightly or not.

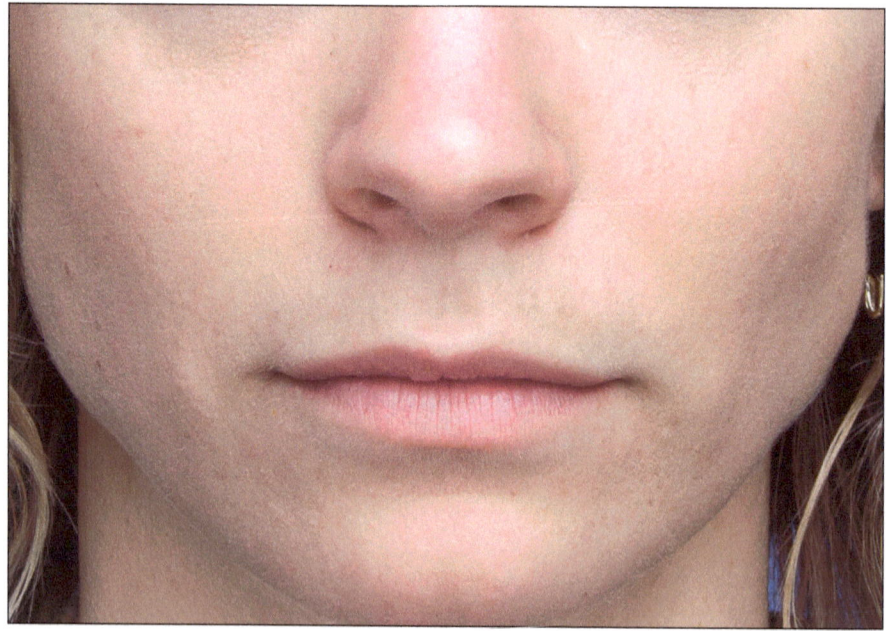

Jaw Muscles that Stick Out

You can then feel those muscles and see how hard they are. The tighter these muscles are the more frequently you do it. People who clench and/or grind only while they are sleeping will have less of a severe tension than someone who clenches and/or grinds heavily during the day or someone who does either/or around the clock.

If you feel the muscles of someone who clenches and/or grinds 24 hours a day, their muscles fibers will be pretty hard to distinguish because they will feel like bone from all the tension.

The other thing to look at with these muscles is if one side sticks out further than the other. If so, that tells you that one side of your mouth is hitting harder than the other side or even that you may only chew on one side.

If you then smile and look at your teeth you may notice that one side is more caved or tilted in than the other side. This will give you an idea of what kind of effect the correct amount of support can make in the mouth.

Many of my patients do not realize that this kind of thing is affecting their face until they look at an old photo of themselves and see that their face is actually becoming square because the muscles in their jaw are sticking out. I can always tell if someone has been clenching and grinding at night as well because they will appear tired more often, and their eyes will often be blood shot because of the strain that is happening in their face while they're sleeping.

Then there are the lines that run from the side of the nostrils to the sides of the mouth. If the lines are on both sides you're most likely looking at a narrow arch.

If you don't treat the root of this problem, which is the structure, and you just treat the symptom with fillers and things of that nature, you are going to be spending a lot of money needlessly.

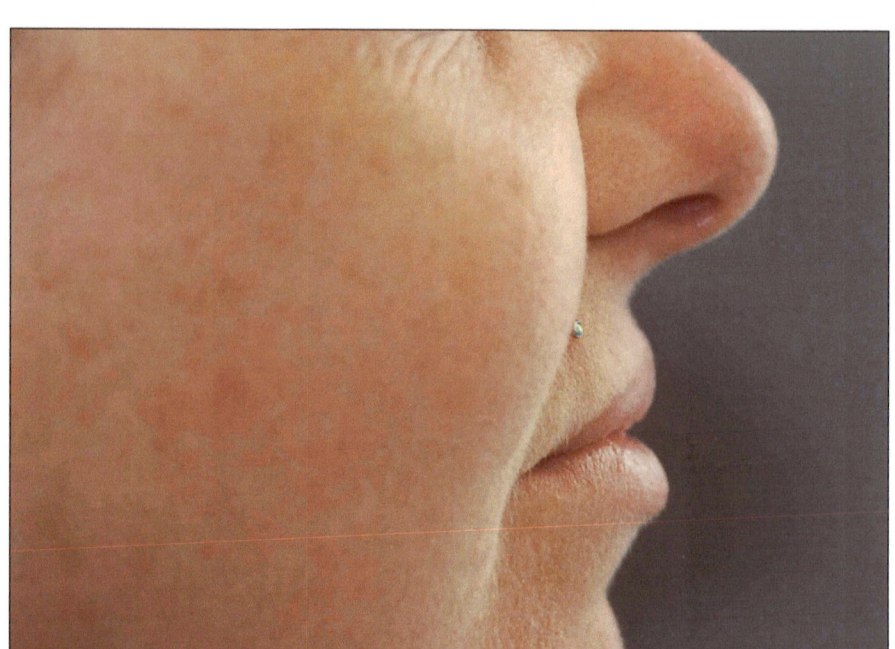

Smile Lines Before

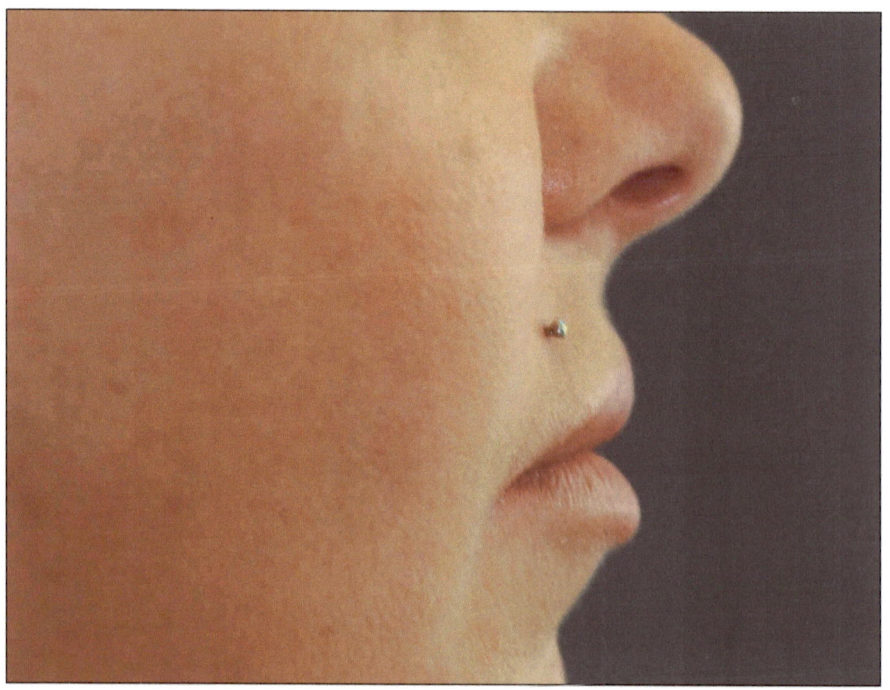

Smile Lines After

It doesn't mean that if someone had their teeth built out to give them support and smooth out these lines that they would never need anything else. It does mean that if you just get the fillers and you don't provide your face with the support it is missing, you will not only have to get procedures done much more frequently, but the problems will continue to get worse, and the lines will continue to get deeper.

The reason these things seem to start showing up very rapidly and become very obvious at a certain age is because the elasticity of the face starts to wane, revealing these problems and imperfections that were hiding. That elasticity can hide all manner of things, and when it starts to go away what's going on underneath the surface will start to become very apparent very quickly.

When I'm examining a patient the key for me is to be sure that if there is a problem in the lower 1/3 of the face I am going to be able to find what is causing that problem on the inside. From that viewpoint I will be able to get a solution for that person that will last a long time because I am making their mouths more structurally sound.

The Next Step

A lot of these things you may be able to see for yourself, but I do recommend, once you are aware of anything, that you seek out a professional who is also familiar with the subject so that they can look at it with an unbiased eye.

A few years ago I treated a relative who flew in from New York to get some work done. He was so happy with what I had done that he went home and told his mother, who had been considering getting some work done herself, that she had to go to me. She thought it seemed unnecessary to fly 5,000 miles to get some dental work done, but her son was so insistent that she decided to at least call me for a recommendation.

She asked me in that conversation what I would do if she was to come out and I explained to her all of the things that I could see that I would address.

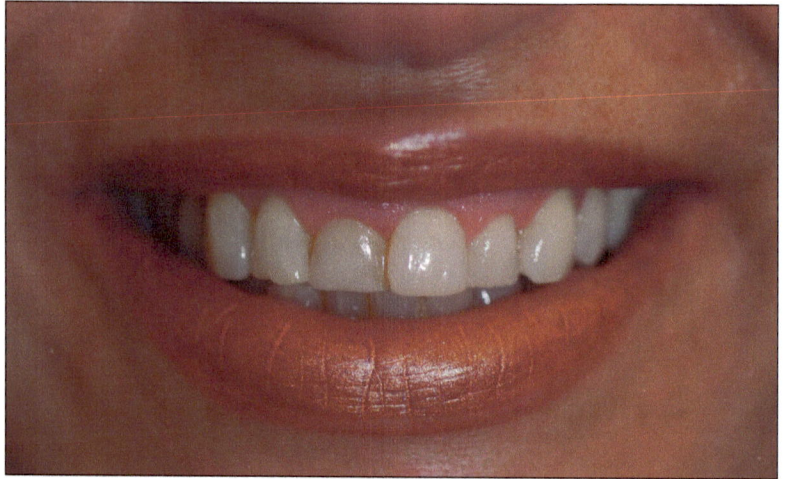

Patient Before

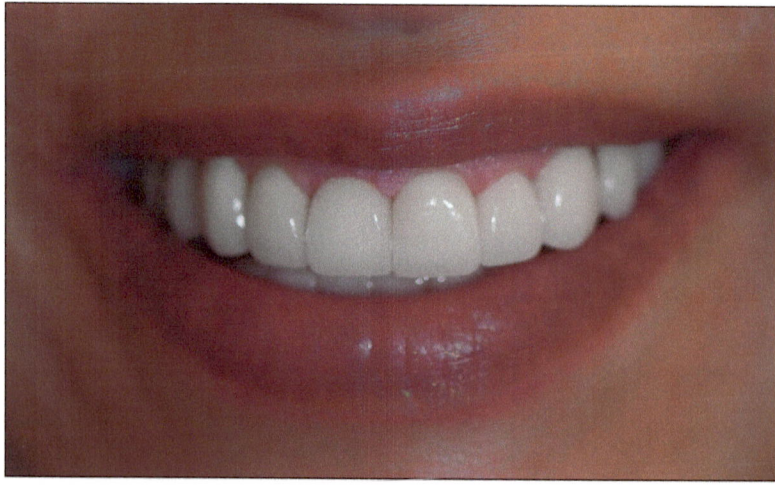

Patient After

She was in shock. She asked me if I was looking at a picture of her or something, and I wasn't. I could just remember these things even though I hadn't seen her in some time. Falling even deeper into disbelief at how I could possibly remember all of those specifics, she became concerned that anyone else would be able to do what I was suggesting.

I told her of two people near her who I believed to be very good, and that she should keep in mind what I had said. If she felt like something was missing, she should call me back and let me know.

A few days later she called me back and said she would be flying out to be treated in my office. I asked her what happened, and she said not only did neither one of the people she saw mention half of what I had said, they also didn't spot the most obvious thing that she had a problem with, which was that her gum on one of her front teeth came down further than the other one.

The dentists she saw are well renowned dentists with established practices in Manhattan, but that doesn't mean that they are going to be aware of the kinds of things I'm talking about here because they are completely new concepts and ways of looking at dentistry. It also doesn't mean that if they do see them they are going to want to take the risk fixing something if they don't have the proper technology to handle it.

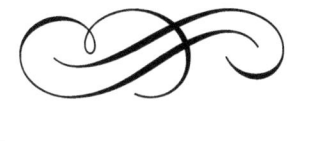

Closing Note

By Caroline Dupuy Heerwagen

I can't tell you what getting to know a dentist has done for my life, and even beyond that I can't tell you how unlikely it would have seemed to me to ever write that sentence down. I dreaded the dentist, hated the dentist even, and now I love my dentist. This is the general consensus with every one of Dr. Maddahi's patients that I've talked to.

During the time I've been around him, I have noticed things about myself I have never considered before, and I can confidently say I never would have. Specifically when I was doing the self-examination with him I saw this.

I sat down with a mirror in my hand as he walked me through each of the steps, and this is when I saw something I had never seen. The right side of my upper lip was more collapsed than the left side. Of course, once I had noticed it I became obsessed with it, but Dr. Maddahi wouldn't give me the answer. He wanted to show me that with everything he was telling me I would be able to figure it out on my own.

So I started paying attention to his exams and looking for the answer when he would break down different cases for me. I wanted to understand how he could see what he saw. I wanted to get it right, because I knew if I could get it right in his eyes, I could get anything right in anyone's.

I don't know why I felt that way, but I did. I think that's what being around the best does to you. It makes you want some piece of that too.

One day after going over a few patients' cases with him, I looked at my teeth and noticed that the right side of them was more crowded and tilted in than the other side. This explained why my lip was collapsed! But it wasn't the whole answer, and I knew it.

I needed to figure out why that side of my teeth was collapsed in order for the answer to be complete. I needed to know the root of the problem, not just the effects it had created.

The next thing I did was feel my jaw near my ear and I could feel right away that though both sides of my face had strained jaw muscles from all the clenching and grinding I do, the muscles protruded more on the right side than the left side. I started asking myself what that could be from. I tried to pay attention to the way I chewed in the days following to see if I was chewing more on one side than the other, but that wasn't it. There was something else.

I thought about this a lot, though I didn't tell Dr. Maddahi I was. I didn't want him to know that I was trying to discover this on my own. One night after getting home, thinking about all the things that I had learned about bad habits, I thought about something I do all the time.

While I was thinking, I was playing with an onlay that sits on the molar on the bottom right side of my jaw with my tongue. That tooth had grown in with no enamel on it, and as a kid, I'd had to get this onlay put on it. I'm sure you can imagine how much I hated it, the girl who screamed bloody murder at dental cleanings. Thankfully for me it's the only porcelain I have in my mouth, as I had never needed a crown or a veneer before or since.

Maybe because it's the only foreign thing in my mouth, I often fiddle with it because it feels funny, and when I caught myself doing it this time it struck me like lightening. I couldn't wait to go in to the office the next day. I walked in the next morning all proud, plopped down in front of him and said, "I figured it out!"

"What did you figure out?" he asked, laughing at the smug expression on my face.

"Why this side of my face is collapsed more than the other side," I explained, like it had been on his mind as much as it had been on mine. He laughed again, shaking his head and waving his hand, gesturing that I should go ahead and tell him.

"It's because of this onlay. My bite was never correct after it was put on, so I clinch that side harder." I sat there for one second to see what his reaction would be. I was dying to know if I'd passed the test, though I had 100% confidence that I was right. I had heard many times since working with him that it's fairly common for dental work like that to change someone's bite and immediately start creating this kind of problem.

"I'm very proud of you. You figured it out," he said.

This may sound funny, but that was probably one of the proudest moments of my life. I laugh even now while writing it because I know it sounds ridiculous, but even this is an example of how he understands people. If he had told me the answer I wouldn't have cared about it. I wouldn't have thought it was a very big deal, because I never think things like that are a very big deal, but because I became fascinated with figuring it out and started noticing the nuances of its effects I wanted to get it fixed right away. I could see it was changing my face, and that it was just going to become more and more apparent as I got older.

This guy actually cares. There were times when I would come in and he would look at me and know that I had been clenching in my sleep the night before because of the color of my eyes. He pays attention.

Here's the simplest way I can put it. Besides the fear of pain there was the fear of being lectured in regard to the dentist for me. Not only do I feel bad about the fact that I don't floss, but I have to hear about what a "bad girl" I am too. I have to hear about how all of my teeth are most certainly going to rot and crumble within the next 6 months. This kind of fear mongering does not encourage me to show up.

Dr. Maddahi does not do this. He never tells his patients they're bad or wrong. He asks the question, "What would you like to improve?" And once he gets the answer he proposes solutions.

I had no idea what I was getting into when I decided to write this book, but I certainly didn't think that a dentist was going to change my life. The perfection he demands in himself rubs off on you, and the dreams and goals I have had for my life have about tripled since being around him. This is what happens. People are transformed. I was transformed. Nancy was transformed. This is an entirely unique person, a completely unique doctor, and even more unique dentist.

www.ingramcontent.com/pod-product-compliance
Lightning Source LLC
Chambersburg PA
CBHW041959150426
43194CB00002B/57